TOTAL FEMALE

Take Charge of Your Sexual Health

Douglas Ginter

Jason Sachman MD

TOTAL FEMALE
Take Charge of Your Sexual Health

"Normal" is nothing more than a cycle on a washing machine.
--Whoopi Goldberg

Take care of your body. It's the only place you have to live. --
Jim Rohn

You were given a body that can stand most anything. It's your mind you have to convince. --Vincent Lombardi

You must begin to think of yourself as becoming the person you want to be. --David Viscott

The time for action is now. It's never too late to do something.
– Carl Sandburg

I dedicate this book to my family. To my wonderful father who died at 55 from prostate cancer, my loving mother at 65 from diabetes related problems, my talented younger brother at 35 from internal demons, and my baby sister at 52 from congestive heart failure. All their untimely passings resulted from the unfortunate combination of their not taking responsibility for their own health and the failure of our current health system to recognize and provide effective treatment for their conditions.

I hope the information in the *Total Female* book helps to make everyone more aware of their potential personal health issues and the easy ways to address them. You have options and nobody can take charge of your health like yourself!

Best wishes to everyone,
—Douglas Ginter

CONTENTS

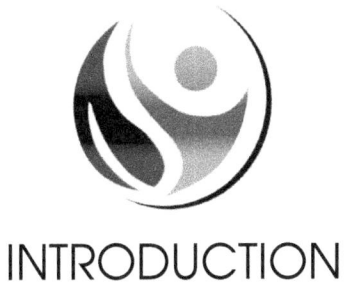

INTRODUCTION

"It just means you are getting old."

"Hormones, darling, can't live with them. Can't live without them."

"Oh every woman deals with that."

Have you heard these phrases from well-meaning loved ones and friends? Then you are probably going through menopause or some other hormonal change, so many people want to pass off as an integral part of life.

However, your body is yours. It and you deserve to be healthy and happy. In addition to overall health, this means sexual health as well. An imbalance in hormones can wreak havoc on your body and cause so many problems that you simply don't feel like having sex anymore. But, that doesn't have to be accepted as the norm. In fact, it isn't. No matter your age, you are still a sexual being and that means your libido shouldn't suffer.

No matter what you have been told and no matter what people think is normal, problems with your hormones and sex drive are not normal. They indicate something is not right in your body and getting everything straightened out is a must.

In the following pages, you will find information about you – a female – from the very basics to the deep down information that will help you get things right with your body.

Are you ready to explore all the things that make you – you? Let's get started…

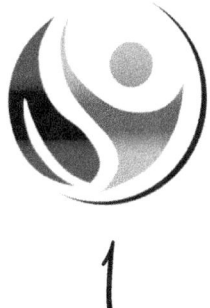

1

Why Am I Reading This Book?

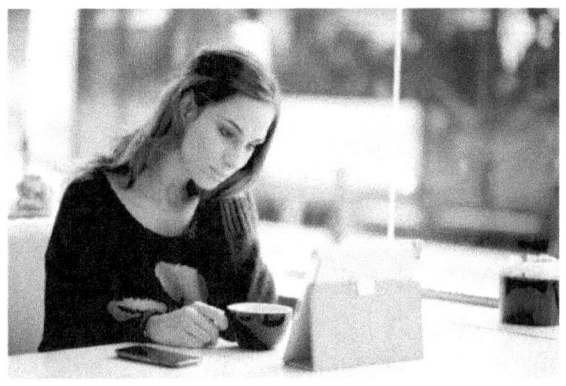

Something is just not right. I know it isn't, but I cannot pinpoint what is actually wrong. I keep telling myself, "Claire, your body changes. Get used to it." But, is my body supposed to change like this? I am only 35! I have completely lost my sex drive. I am intimate with my husband, but I just do not enjoy it anymore. That's not the only problem in that department either. There's the dryness, which actually makes sex painful. I feel like if things keep going the way they are, my husband and I will start drifting apart.

It's too embarrassing to talk about though, so I haven't told my husband or my doctor. Maybe it's all in my head, I think.

But, it's not. I know it isn't.

Because, the sex issues aren't my only problems. I am tired all the time, and I mean ALL the time. I can get a good night's sleep and feel exhausted the next day. I can't think straight either. How many times have I heard "Earth to Claire" lately? Too many to count.

What's wrong with me? I know this can't be normal.

Claire is facing the same type of challenges that women all over the country, and all over the globe for that matter, experience every day. And, no, they aren't normal. Claire's instincts are right. But, just as she has no idea what is going on with her body, millions of other women do not either. You may be one of them. Hopefully, that is why you are reading this book.

Changes in Sexual Health

The truth is that changes in sexual health can occur for a variety of different reasons. All of those reasons eventually trace back to hormones. Women will experience these changes, especially after certain events, such as:

- Childbirth

- Menopause

- Illness that leads to hormone imbalance

- Starting a new type of prescription medication

All too often, people chalk up these changes to a "natural part of life." Women are told to "suck it up and deal with it." That is, unfortunately, the majority view, but it doesn't have to be the reality for you or any other woman.

Did you find yourself nodding in agreement when you read Claire's story? Are you experiencing symptoms like hers?

"If you are having these problems, you are not alone. The three most common sexual issues are:

- Not being in the mood for sex

- Trouble becoming aroused (vaginal dryness) and having orgasms

- Pain during sex or sexual activity" (Sexual Difficulties)

While millions of women deal with these issues, none of them have to, since there are treatments available to help lessen their effects.

Sexual Health and Aging

Women who are approaching or in the midst of menopause are often told there is nothing they can do to change their situation. The reasons for issues in sexual health during this change of life are hormones or imbalances in the natural hormones the woman's body requires.

While the symptoms of menopause have long been thought of as unavoidable, this is not true. There are treatments, which we will discuss later. That may be why you are reading this book. Perhaps you have experienced symptoms such as:

Irregular periods	Vaginal dryness
Hot flashes	Irritability
Night sweats	Extreme fatigue
Memory problems	Weight gain

Those types of symptoms are considered "normal" when women go through menopause, but why should they be? When you understand more about your body and your own sexual health, you will be armed with the knowledge you need to understand how you can get your life back.

Understanding Your Body

How well do you actually understand your body? Do you know what it is trying to say to you? Often, women overlook the warning signs their bodies are giving, or they have a feeling that something "isn't quite right" and then try to push that feeling away.

Understanding your sexual health is an important step in your journey to getting back to the life you want. Can you think back to your teenage years when you took a sex education class? How much do you actually remember?

While it may seem like a given, it is vital that you refresh your mind on how your body works. Learn who you are physically, because the more you know about your own body, the more you can read signs that something isn't quite right or "normal."

So, why are you reading this book? Whatever reason you may have, you are reading this book because you want to be prepared and knowledgeable about your body.

In the following pages, we will discuss everything in detail, starting with getting to know your body and then moving on to topics like:

- Where your sexual desire actually comes from;

- How men can actually experience lack of desire as well;

- The important role of hormones in your body;

- The problems women face with their sexual health;

- Treatments available for those problems;

- Reversing the physical effects of aging, and

- Understanding stem cell banking.

This book isn't about anyone else. It is about you, your body, and your sexual health. So, read it as a love story – a love story that will help you understand *you* on a whole different level. Changes in sexual health don't have to be tolerated. Are you ready to find out why?

One last note to keep in mind: it doesn't matter your age. This book isn't just for women facing menopause. Yes, many changes in sexual health do happen during that time, but women of any age can experience the types of hormone imbalances that lead to problems. So, you don't have to pass an age test to learn from these pages. It doesn't matter if you are 21, 71, or anywhere in between. This book is still written for you.

Before we delve into the deep and more advanced material, we should start by going back to the basics. It takes a basic understanding of your body for you to understand the things that could possibly be going wrong with it. In the next chapter, we will revisit a "high school health class". We will discuss the basics of your body and how your reproductive organs work. If you already know the material in chapter two, then consider it a refresher of sorts. It doesn't hurt to go back to the very basic information and remind yourself of things you may have forgotten or taken for granted over the years.

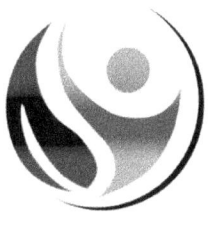

2

My Body

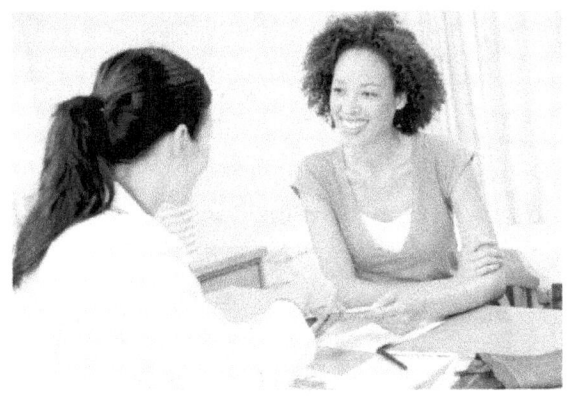

I always thought I knew my body pretty well. I mean it is my body; it would be kind of strange if I didn't know how it works. But, I guess I didn't understand it quite as well as I thought. I knew I needed hormones. I knew they had something to do with my fertility. I had no idea they had an effect on ALL of my sexual health. When things just weren't quite right for me – about six months after having a baby – I decided to go see the doctor. I wasn't sure why so suddenly I was so

dry...down there. I really thought that I knew everything there was to know about my body.

Then, sitting there in the doctor's office, I heard them call "Jeanine, are you ready?"

It was right then that I began to wish I had paid a little more attention in my college anatomy class because I really didn't know as much as I thought.

Once my doctor explained things to me, it all started to make sense, and I certainly have gotten things sorted out now, but I cannot help but think if I had known my body a little better, then I wouldn't have waited so long to see the physician. That would have meant less time I spent dealing with those problems.

How well do you actually know your body? How much do you remember from classes you have taken or research you have done on your own? You live in your body every single day, so it's very easy to take it for granted.

However, your physical being is a complicated process. It works in ways that are hard for anyone to fully understand. Every organ, every cell, every part of your body works together. When one thing doesn't work quite right, you can be affected in ways you couldn't expect.

So, before we can truly delve into your sexual health, we need to talk about your body. You may read this whole chapter and already know everything, but then again, you may read it and think "wow...I didn't know that's how that works!". Let's look at two main categories: your breasts and your reproductive organs.

Keep in mind that your reproductive health and your sexual health are interwoven together. A problem with one can lead to issues with the other. That's why it's so important that you understand all of the organs that make you female.

Breasts

Your breasts can be a source of life, since they are designed specifically to provide nourishment to a newborn baby. They can be a source of pain at certain times of the month. They certainly lend to a woman's sexuality and be a source of pleasure.

The female breast can be different sizes and shapes, but they are all made up of the same tissues. How much do you know about them?

> "The breast is the tissue overlying the chest (pectoral) muscles. Women's breasts are made of specialized tissue that produces milk (glandular tissue) as well as fatty tissue. The amount of fat determines the size of the breast." (Women's Health, 2012)

That can be a little confusing, so let's back up for a second. Yes, the layer of fat near the surface of the breast does determine its size, but that doesn't necessarily mean the amount of fat on the rest of the body correlates with the amount in the breasts.

However, when women do gain weight, they will also gain fat in the breasts. That's why your bra sizes can change through the years.

Underneath the fatty tissue layer, your breasts include an intricate system that allows them to produce milk when needed. There are between 15 and 20 lobules within your breasts that allow milk to be produced. These lobules open into ducts that connect together and lead to the nipple. Other tissues found within the breasts include:

Lymph Nodes	Blood Vessels
Lymph Vessels	Ligaments
Nerves	Connective Tissues

Your breasts have their shape because of the connective tissues that hold everything together. Every woman, and that means EVERY woman, has a different shape to their breasts. There is no "normal".

Why Do Breasts Get Sore?

I started my period when I was 12 years old and I developed breasts soon after. I am not particularly well-endowed or anything. I am a modest 34B. That's nothing to sneeze at I guess. But, here is the problem. Every month, about a week before my period, my breasts get very sore.

They get so sore that I am not comfortable exercising, even with a sturdy sports bra. I hate it when they are bumped and any "attention" from my husband is a big no-no during that time. It hurts too much!

I thought this was normal, because I read somewhere that all women's breasts get sore before their period. Then, I was commiserating with one of my friends and she said it didn't sound right. "Yours don't get sore?" I asked? Her response: "Well, they feel a little strange, but nothing like you are talking about!"

That's when I realized I was dealing with something that wasn't normal. That's when I decided to go to the doctor and I found out my hormones were out of whack.

———————————

There are a few different reasons why your breasts can become sore. They include the following:

• Cyclic Pain – This refers to the pain you feel in your breasts just before your period. Women even in peri-menopause can experience this type of cycle pain. Within a week before your menstrual period, you go through PMS symptoms. Your body is releasing two main types of hormones, and they actually cause you to retain water. That includes in your breasts. This stretches and irritates the breast tissues causing soreness, swelling, and lumps.

• Pregnancy -- You will experience soreness due to the flood of hormones going through your body. Then, as you get closer to your due date, your breasts will become sore and swollen as the lobules begin producing milk, in anticipation for the baby.

• Other Sources – Other things can cause breast pain as well. These include hormone imbalances, medications like birth control and even certain antidepressants, infection, injury, cysts, and muscle strain.

The breast tissues are sensitive, and as a result, can experience all sorts of pains like sharp stabbing, burning, aching, and more.

The Erogenous Zone

On the outside of your breasts, you have nipples. Of course, they are designed specifically to feed babies. However, they also contribute to sexual health and sexuality. You already know that your nipples, surrounded by the areola (dark skin around the nipple) are an erogenous zone. But, do you know why? We are going to have to delve into science to answer that question.

The Journal of Sexual Medicine published a study in 2011 explains this. According to the study,

> "Using functional magnetic resonance imaging (fMRI), researchers noted which brain areas become active when women touch various parts of their bodies. The genital-sensing brain areas in women roughly correspond to the same areas in men, but the nipple finding was a surprise.
>
> 'My speculation is that this could be the basis for many women saying that nipple stimulation is erotogenic, because it stimulates the same area as the genitals.'" (Pappas, 2011)

This means that when your breasts are touched, the same part of the brain goes to work as if you are involved in sexual conduct. That's why they are just as important to your sexual health as other parts of your body and they are very much an erogenous zone.

Here is something important to remember, as it has become a source of urban legend in modern society. Breast size itself is not correlated in any way to a woman's sexuality or her ability to experience pleasure from her breasts being caressed. Women have differences in sensation based totally on their hormones and brain, and it has nothing to do with the actual size of their breasts. So, to put it simply, a woman with small breasts could very well have extremely sensitive breasts, to the point that she is able to climax from touching them alone and a woman with very large breasts may have little sensitivity at all, and vice versa.

So the myth that women with bigger breasts are more sexual is just that…a myth.

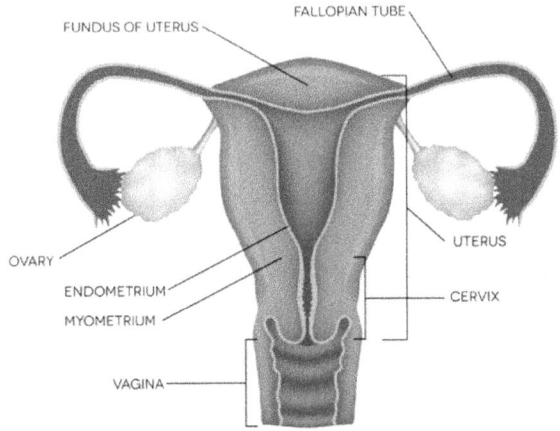

Female Reproductive Organs

The next step in understanding your body is to know more about your reproductive organs. Most of us have a basic idea of how they work, but we don't know all of the important details. However, you can't just know the basics. After all, it is your body and knowing what's going on inside is extremely important. Most of your reproductive system is located inside of your body for a few different reasons: this way, your body is capable of carrying a baby, and to ensure your organs are less exposed to bacteria and infection.

To look at things in detail, let's discuss the external reproductive system (genitals), separately from the internal organs.

External

Your external anatomy is designed to protect your internal organs and it is designed to offer you sexual pleasure when you are aroused. Let's talk about four different parts.

• Labia Majora

The labia majora translates exactly to "large lips" and are the flaps of skin located on each side of the vaginal opening. They are capable of completely coming together to create protection for the internal organs. They are also the portions that are covered with hair.

Here's something you may not know about your outer or larger labia: they contain sweat glands. Yes, that means you sweat down there. You probably already knew that, but now you know this is 100% normal.

The labia majora can be shaped differently from one woman to the next and there is no "norm" with how they look. Additionally, when you become sexually aroused, they will swell and become more sensitive.

• Labia Minora

Translating exactly to "small lips", the labia minora are two flaps of skin that are located within the labia majora. They surround the vaginal and urethral openings. The smaller labia may or may not be very visible, unless you are sexually aroused.

The labia minora are often a concern for women, since they can look so different from one woman to the next. There are even plastic surgeries designed to give these small lips a more aesthetically pleasing look. However, it is perfectly natural for women to have completely different looking labia minora from one another.

• Bartholin Glands

Located on each side of the vaginal opening, the Bartholin glands provide lubrication to the labia. You cannot see these glands and you probably were not even aware they existed.

In some cases, the glands may become backed up or blocked and this can lead to painful cysts. These cysts may look scary, but they are generally harmless and very easy to treat.

• Clitoris

Finally we have the big finish … the show stopper… the clitoris, often simply referred to as "the clit". This small button of flesh is located in front of the vaginal and urethral opening and at where the labia minora meet in the front. It is surrounded by a semicircular "hood" of tissue that will usually retract when the clitoris becomes swollen during sexual arousal.

This one little spot has as many nerve endings as found in the whole head of a man's penis and it is extremely sensitive. In fact, the majority of women are only able to climax through clitoral stimulation, so it does play a very important role in your sexual health.

Because the clitoris is so sensitive, it can be uncomfortable for some woman during direct stimulation. In fact, some women even refer to this type of touch as painful and they prefer indirect stimulation. The sensitivity of the clitoris varies from one woman to the next. There is no norm in this case either. You may or may not be able to handle direct stimulation. You may or may not be able to climax solely from stimulation to the clitoris. No matter the case, no matter what seems to work for you, you are as normal as the next woman.

That's all of your external reproductive parts, and they all work together to protect your internal organs, to ensure reproduction is possible, and to give you sexual pleasure. However, when they malfunction in some way, you can lose that pleasure altogether. For example, if the labia majora and minora are not properly lubricated and you are experiencing vaginal dryness, then they can become irritated and painful.

We are going to discuss various problems that could stand in the way of your sexual health later in this book. For now, let's move on to taking a look at your internal reproductive parts.

Internal

Your internal organs are designed specifically to ensure you are able to carry and give birth to a baby. Let's look at those four parts now:

- Ovaries

  You have two ovaries. They are located to the sides of the uterus and they perform two functions. One of those is to produce eggs that will travel down the Fallopian tubes and into the uterus. The second function of the ovaries is to secrete estrogen and progesterone and a small amount of testosterone.

  When you go through menopause, your ovaries eventually stop producing estrogen.

  Ovaries generally trade off which one produces an egg each month. That's why it is completely possible to get pregnant even if you have only one functioning ovary. There are also cases when both ovaries produce an egg in a given month and this can result in fraternal twins.

- Fallopian Tubes

  When an ovary releases an egg, the ova then travels down the fallopian tubes. They are located on each side of the uterus and they are connected to the uterus, but not the ovaries themselves. Instead, they contain small hair like follicles that catch the egg and pull it into the tube.

  When a woman gets pregnant, the conception actually occurs within the fallopian tubes.

Once the egg is fertilized, it travels the rest of the way down the tubes and implants within the uterus. On some occasions, the egg may attach inside the tubes and result in something called an ectopic pregnancy. This type of pregnancy cannot be carried to term and often results in loss of that fallopian tube altogether. Keep in mind, that this doesn't mean the woman will be infertile, since she will have another functioning ovary and fallopian tube.

• Uterus

The easiest way to envision the uterus is to think of an upside down pear. It is wider at the top and it culminates in a narrow portion called the cervix. The uterus itself is called the corpus and though it is very small naturally, it can expand immensely to carry a child to full term.

The cervix at the end of the uterus is a donut shaped organ with a small opening in the center. That opening will expand during labor to allow the baby to pass through. The rest of the time, it remains very small and only has enough room for menstrual blood and sperm to pass through.

• Vagina

Finally, you have the vagina, which is a canal that connects your internal reproductive organs and the external tissues. It is often referred to as the birth canal since it is the area in which the baby travels out of the body during birth. At one end of the vagina is the opening through the labia. At the other end is the cervix.

"The vagina resembles a deflated tube that's only 2 to 4 inches long and three-fourths of an inch wide. However, the vagina is lined with ringed muscular ridges so that it can expand when necessary, such as during intercourse or childbirth. During sexual intercourse for example, the vagina swells to approximately 4 to 8 inches in length and 2.5 inches in width." (Edmonds)

There are a couple of things we need to discuss about the vagina in detail. To begin with, only the bottom portion of tissue within the vagina actually has nerve endings. So, the length of a man's penis really doesn't matter when it comes to sensation for the woman.

The second thing to understand is the hymen. This very thin skin tissue covers a part of the vaginal opening when a woman is born. Over time, the hymen can become torn for numerous reasons, like using tampons or riding a bike. If a woman's hymen doesn't tear during her first sexual intercourse, this does not mean she was not a virgin. It simply means it tore earlier for other reasons.

Finally, there is the much argued idea of the G-spot, which is a sensitive area of tissue about halfway up the inside, front wall of the vagina. Many people do not think it exists. However, many women are able to achieve climax from the stimulation of this area. If you are unfamiliar with it, it is easy to find. As mentioned, about a few inches within the vagina on the front wall (toward your belly button), you will find a bumpy patch of tissue that feels somewhat raised and different from surrounding tissues.

That's the gist of how your reproductive organs work. Chances are there were some things you learned in this chapter and that will give you a better understanding of how your body works.

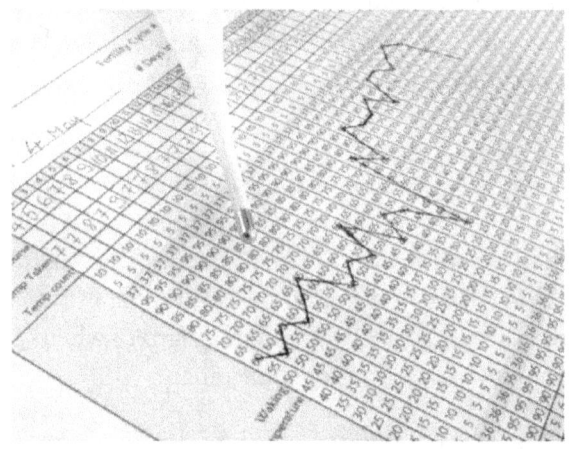

The Menstrual Cycle

Let's get down to the basics of the menstrual cycle because you may not thoroughly understand everything your body goes through during the month. This cycle is controlled completely by hormones. That's why some women, who suffer from hormonal imbalances, may suffer also from irregular periods and confusing cycles.

> "The menstrual cycle is a series of changes a woman's body goes through to prepare for pregnancy. About once a month, the uterus grows a new lining (endometrium) to get ready for a fertilized egg. When there is no fertilized egg to start a pregnancy, the uterus sheds its lining. This is the monthly menstrual bleeding

that women have from their early teen years until menopause, around age 50." (Normal Menstrual Cycle)

Here are a few facts about the cycle that you may not know:

• It starts from the first day you bleed and ends the first day you bleed the next time.

• The average cycle is 28 days, but it can vary from one woman to the next.

• A longer or shorter cycle doesn't mean there is anything wrong.

• The bleeding portion of the cycle generally lasts five days, but can vary anywhere between three and seven days, without being considered abnormal.

Your menstrual cycle, as mentioned, is completely controlled by hormones, so let's talk about what actually goes on within your body when hormones trigger action.

To begin with, two parts of your brain, the pituitary gland and hypothalamus, send signals to your ovaries. These signals are sent through two different types of hormones: estrogen and progesterone. When estrogen is released, this signals the uterus to begin building up the lining in preparation for the egg. The progesterone causes the ovary to release an egg on about day 15 of your cycle.

If the egg is not fertilized, then both estrogen and progesterone will drop near the end of the cycle and this signals the uterus to break down the lining. This is when you have your period. These changes in hormone levels will trigger other changes in your body:

- Premenstrual Phase – This occurs just before the period and you may experience weight gain and bloating due to water retention, tender and sore breasts, acne, lack of energy, abdominal cramps, anxiety, and even depression. This time is often referred to as PMS, and when the condition actually interrupts a woman's daily life, this could be a sign that she suffers from PMDD, or premenstrual dysmorphic disorder.

- Menstrual Phase – During your period, you may experience cramps, constipation or even diarrhea, nausea, a feeling of tiredness, and even irritability.

Every woman is different and they may or may not experience these symptoms or changes in their body. Some women are lucky enough to never experience a single menstrual cramp, while for other women, the pain is almost debilitating.

Problems that Affect the Cycle

Women who have irregular periods may be experiencing hormonal imbalances because hormones are not sending the right signals to the uterus and ovaries. There are other factors that can change the cycle as well, including:

- Menopause and Peri-Menopause

- Weight Gain or Extreme Weight Loss

- Birth Control Pills

- Stress

- Extreme Exercise

Of course, pregnancy will interrupt the cycle as well. Generally, teens who are just experiencing puberty, as well as women who are experiencing menopause, will deal with irregular cycles, heavy bleeding, and other problems simply because there are various changes to the hormones themselves. We will discuss hormones to a greater extent later in this book.

Now you have a much better idea of how your body works, what it does to ensure you are fertile and what actually forms your sexuality. This is the first step to taking charge of your sexual health. In the next chapter, we will discuss sexual desire and arousal itself, because there are several things that affect this, including hormones, the brain, and the body. It's important that you understand what actually triggers sexual desire, so that you will also be able to understand when something isn't quite right.

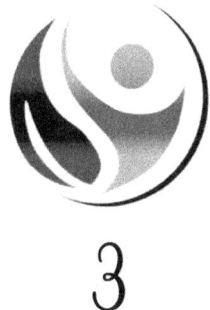

3

Understanding Sexual Desire

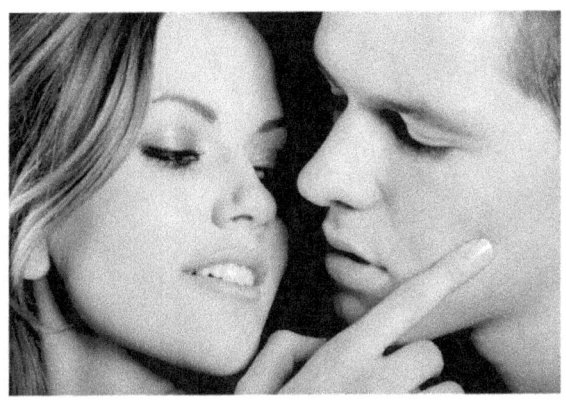

There are quite a few different names for sexual desire, including libido, sex drive, sexual motivation, passion, turned on, horny, randy, or frisky, depending on who is actually using the term. Sexual desire is a biological need or drive and it is a part of being human being. Generally, a person experiences sexual desire, which makes them hunger for sexual activity. A lack of sexual desire and enjoyment from sex, can be an indicator that something is may be wrong.

When you get "turned on" several things happen within your body all at once. Women have different feelings

27

and reactions, but it is very important that you understand your own body. That way, if something changes, you will notice it. So, let's begin by talking about how your body changes when you feel sexual arousal and desire.

Physical Reaction in Men and Women

There are certain parts of your brain that are triggered when you experience sexual arousal. We already mentioned this when we discussed your breasts. When these portions of your brain are triggered, they begin to tell the rest of your body what to do. This includes:

- The nipples become hard and erect. The breasts tend to swell.

- Blood flow increases to your genitals, which this leads to more sensitivity and swollen tissue.

- The vagina begins to lubricate itself.

- The clitoris swells and becomes harder.

- The muscles near the vaginal opening tend to tighten.

Climax or orgasm occurs when sexual desire culminates by stimulation. For some women who are experiencing hormonal imbalance, a lack of desire, a lack of sexual pleasure, and inability to orgasm are common issues. We will discuss theseissues later in this chapter.

The reaction in men is similar to what women experience since blood flow is concentrated in the genital area. During sexual stimulation, the increased blood flow to the penis causes it to become erect and hard.

The Brain's Role

Let's talk about the brain in further detail. Many people refer to it as the ultimate sex organ for good reason. It does play a huge role in your sexual desire. There is a section of your brain that is often referred to as the pleasure center. It reacts to all types of pleasure including laughter, happiness, and of course, sexual desire. It also includes something referred to as a reward circuit. In other words, when you experience pleasure, like sexual activity, your brain rewards you by making you feel even better.

When you go experience sexual desire, several parts of your brain are affected, including:

- The pituitary gland releases endorphins and oxytocin, which make you feel good and feel less pain. This increases trust and bonding feelings, and that is why many people feel much closer to another person after having sexual intercourse. Keep in mind that the pituitary gland plays a part in releasing the hormones required by your body for your monthly cycle.

- The cerebellum, which controls muscle function, is also triggered during sexual intercourse, and this helps to achieve orgasm.

- The Amygdala is a part of the brain that helps to control emotions. During sexual desire, this part of your brain triggers two different kinds of feelings: those of happiness and those of a sexual desire.

- The nucleus accumbens and the ventral tegmental area are responsible for releasing dopamine (the feel good hormone) during sexual arousal and the actual act of sexual intercourse.

A study about the brain's role in sexual desire was completed in the early 2000's by a group of people in the Netherlands at the University of Groningen. This study covered men and women, but it focused especially on the effect of sexual desire in women. Here are a few of the findings from this study:

- A region of the brain called the lateral orbitofrontal cortex (the reason center) of the brain shuts down during orgasm. Essentially, you really do lose control when you climax.

- In women, the PAG, a part of the brain stem, reacts. This is the part of your brain that controls your fight or flight mechanism. Essentially, in women, fear is lessened and the fight or flight reaction is deactivated. For women to experience true sexual pleasure, this has to happen, so that they can feel totally relaxed.

- In women, a part of the cortex that controls pain is also triggered, indicating that pain and pleasure are intertwined during sexual activity and desire. (Freeman)

For women, sexual desire doesn't really come from spontaneous attraction or need. Instead, it is signaled by specific reasons, like an expression of love, an emotional connection with another individual, a need to feel validation, to meet a partner's sexual needs, and to feel powerful.

Hormones and Their Effect

We will talk about the hormones as a whole in a later chapter, but right now, let's talk about those hormones that are directly connected with sexual desire. You have something in your body called androgens, and they are directly linked to your sex drive.

Understanding Androgens

These Androgens are created and secreted by the ovaries and adrenal glands and they are a group of different hormones, the most well-known being Testosterone. Men have more Androgens in their body than women, but this doesn't necessarily affect the power of sex drive. In fact, because women are much more sensitive to the Androgens, they react very differently. Quite simply, women don't need as many androgens to feel sexual arousal. In fact, you have a very specifically designed hormonal system that keeps your body from developing too many androgens. That's important, because if you do start producing too many, some of the symptoms can include:

- Excess hair growth, especially on the face;

- More muscular development;

- Redistribution of body fat, and

- In serious cases, the higher risk for ovarian cancer.

Your body properly regulates the amount of androgens in your body, unless that is, you have a hormonal imbalance.

Estrogen and the Sex Drive

Androgens aren't the only hormones that affect your sexual desire. Estrogen makes you more sensitive and creates the right environment within your vaginal tissue, so that you enjoy sex more. Estrogen is responsible for the elasticity and lubrication of the vagina, and an imbalance of this hormone can lead to sexual discomfort.

While scientists are unclear on how estrogen directly affects sex drive, what they do know is because of estrogen, women can enjoy sex more.

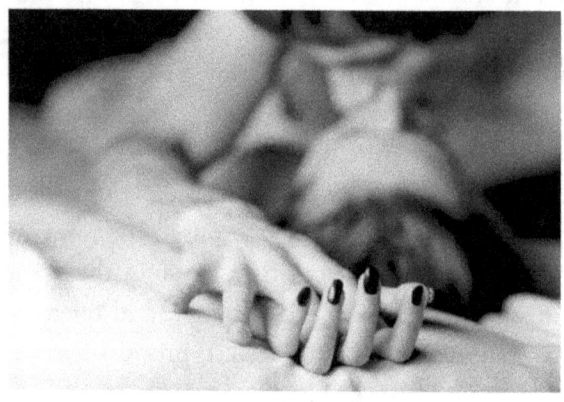

Let's Talk about Pheromones

While pheromones aren't the same types of hormones we have been discussing, it is important that we discuss them in connection with the chemistry of sexual desire.

Every day, your body sends out pheromones, or compounds, that actually travel by air. One of the biggest fuels for sexual arousal is your reaction to others pheromones.

"Pheromones, unlike most other hormones are ectohormones –act outside the body of the individual secreting them – they impact a behavior on another individual. Hormones typically only affect the individual secreting them. Pheromones are secreted to trigger many types of behaviors that include:

- Alarm

- Following food

- Sexual arousal

- Territorial behaviors

- Mother and child bonding

- Intimidation." (What Are Pheromones? Do Humans Have Pheromones?, 2011)

Have you ever heard someone say they were afraid because they got a fear "vibe" off of someone else? This is likely due to pheromones. We secrete them constantly without even knowing it and they basically tell others what to do. This includes sexual attraction. Essentially, when someone is sexually attracted to someone else, before they even know that person, pheromones likely play a big role in this.

That's not all either. Your sexual arousal can be triggered by the other person's arousal too. When they breathe hard, experience a faster heartbeat, and release more arousal pheromones, then your body will react to accordingly.

What Goes on in My Body During Sexual Arousal?

Sexual arousal is multifaceted and very intricate. There is much more going on in your body than you may have ever realized. Let's talk about some internal things that are happening. Generally, there is a specific time frame of intense sexual arousal. It usually only lasts a few moments, but it can go on longer. During that time, here are some of the things going on inside your body:

- Your pulse quickens.

- Blood flow to the genitals increases, as we already mentioned.

- The blood flow to your genitals, like the labia minora, can cause color change. They may darken, turn red or even turn a purple color.

- Your skin on your chest and face may become mottled (often referred to as the sex flush).

- You find that your senses are heightened and you are much more aware of everything around you.

- Your muscles focus on sexual activity.

There is a myth floating around about sexual desire, and it is very unfortunate. Many people assume that sexual activity and desire is only for younger people. In fact, they think that people completely lose their yearning to have sexual intercourse when they become older, but that is simply not true. Despite menopause and despite the changes in the body, sexual desire and intercourse are an important part of a woman's body and needs for her whole life, no matter her age.

Loss of sexual desire during menopause, or at different times in life due to changes in hormones, is not a requirement. It is actually a problem that needs to be corrected. So, let's talk about that.

What Happened to My Sexual Desire?

I have always enjoyed sex. In fact, when my husband and I got married, the old phrase that had something to do with bunnies held true. I had a strong sex drive and getting turned on was never an issue for me.

Even after I turned 40, I got great joy out of sex. I was amazed when some of my friends complained because their husbands wanted it more often than they did. I kept thinking, "Really? I mean that sounds like something to make you happy!" It blew my mind that women discussed different excuses they could use to get out of sex. Then, here I was feeling like some type of nympho.

Something happened though. I don't really know what it was, since I haven't even started going through menopause yet. I just stopped feeling sexual desire. I couldn't get turned on. It was so frustrating! I wanted sex. I wanted to be turned on. I wanted to jump my husband's bones when he came in from work, but I just didn't feel it.

This is not the life I was used to. I hated it. What was happening to me? That's a question I finally discussed with my doctor, because it became such a source of frustration. I found out it really wasn't normal. I wasn't just getting older. I was losing my sexual desire for a reason, and once that reason was uncovered, my husband and I could get back to acting like bunnies.

Women who are going through menopause and even those in the years leading up to this change of life, will have wildly varying hormone levels. This can cause a whole variety of different sexual side effects, but that doesn't mean they are normal. It doesn't mean that going through menopause is the death of sexual desire.

Additionally, some of the body changes associated with menopause, that affect sexual desire, include:

- The vaginal area could become thinner and that means it may feel more irritation.

- The vagina will not produce as much lubrication.

- The thickness of the vaginal walls may decrease.

- The clitoris may become less sensitive.

Because of all this, a woman may find sexual intercourse painful or uncomfortable and that can directly lead to a decrease in sexual arousal. Essentially, if you can't enjoy sex, you probably find it hard to even get turned on by the idea of it!

Additionally, orgasm itself, may become uncomfortable or extremely difficult to achieve. There are a few reasons for this. The muscles that contract during orgasm may become weaker, or, the orgasmic contractions in the uterus actually may become painful. This can certainly contribute to lack of sexual desire. You may be afraid to have sex or you may worry that you won't enjoy it. The stress of this worry can have a direct impact on your ability to get turned on.

Explanations

Here is a quick rundown of other things that can directly affect a woman's sexual desire or libido.

- Medical conditions including cancer, diabetes, neurological conditions, arthritis and coronary artery disease.

- Prescription medications including antidepressants and anti-seizure medications

- Drinking alcohol or using illicit drugs

- Exhaustion and stress

- Surgery on genital parts

- Post pregnancy hormonal changes

- Menopausal hormonal changes

- Depression and other mental health problems

- Poor body image and low self-esteem

- Sexual abuse in the past

- Unresolved conflicts with the spouse

- Lack of connected feeling with the spouse or partner

- Infidelity in the marriage or another type of trust breach

The female sexual anatomy is very intricate and detailed. Any number of things can negatively affect it. Hormones play a massive role, and as women face menopause or deal with other hormonal changes, they will lose the hormones that are directly connected with desire.

The good news is that there are things you can do, and we will focus on that soon. It is completely possible to grow older and still enjoy sex. The very idea that you should stop enjoying sex is rather ludicrous. You just need to know what may have changed in your body and what needs to be done about it.

I Still Have It, Why Doesn't He?

I know that lots of women lose their sex drive as they get older. I have heard it from some of my friends who are going through menopause. It's not really a surprise when a woman just doesn't feel like sex anymore, but what has happened in my marriage is really confusing.

I still want sex. I still love sex and I most certainly get turned on. I am not the problem. In fact, my sex drive is ready and raring to go. No, it's not me. He is the one who doesn't have it anymore.

For a while, I was convinced it must be something about me. Maybe he just was not attracted to me anymore. After all, I am 43 and I have started to get those lovely little wrinkles around my eyes. My breasts are sagging a little. Yes, I thought it was me. I just wasn't attractive and my husband couldn't get turned on—that's what I thought, but it wasn't the truth.

In fact, my husband told me regularly just how attracted he was to me. He pointed out that I still had a sexy butt and that he thought my smile was the sexiest thing he had ever seen. But...he just didn't want sex anymore.

I tried all sorts of stuff: I wore naughty lingerie, bought new "toys", and even suggested we watch porn together. We still had sex from time to time, but things weren't what they used to be.

It took some urging to talk my husband into going to the doctor, but eventually he did and found out he had low testosterone. Since he has been on hormone replacement therapy, things have revved back up in the bedroom. I have to say, it's pretty awesome.

What happens when you still enjoy a healthy level of sexual desire, but your husband doesn't? It's not the norm or what most people expect, but it does happen. There are lots of reasons why men may lose their sexual desire, and one of them is most certainly loss of hormones. Androgens are important to a man's sexuality too, so when there aren't enough of them in his body, this can cause him to lose his desire for sexual intercourse.

This can be a rather difficult situation, especially if a woman is dealing with a poor self-image. The woman doesn't think she looks good and when her husband doesn't want sex that often, she assumes that it is because of her. That's exactly what the woman in the story above did. However, it is very important to understand there are reasons, both physical and emotional, that can lead to a loss of sexual desire.

Explanations

Let's take a quick look at the various reasons why a man may lose his sexual desire as well:

- Mental concerns, such as anxiety or depression

- Prescription medications, which may inhibit a man's sex drive

- Illness and other medical conditions

- Low testosterone levels

Men can lose their sex drive for many of the same reasons that women do, even though they don't go through menopause. That's why it is equally important for men to consider hormone replacement therapy, as loss of testosterone may be the culprit for a decreasing sex drive.

People tend to blame hormones for everything – headaches, hot flashes, moodiness, being snappish, and even forgetting to turn off the coffee pot. It's true that a hormonal imbalance can be a factor in these types of symptoms. That's not all though. A hormonal imbalance is the number one reason why women and men lose their sex drive. A loss of libido should never be considered normal either. It's only through an understanding of how sexual desire works, that you can see the things that could be going wrong with it.

Now that we have discussed sexual desire and you can see how it is directly connected to your hormones, it is time to talk about hormones themselves in detail. The more you understand hormones and all of the ways they affect your body, the better you can prepare yourself to find the right treatment. This will ensure that you won't continue having to deal with the negative side effects of a hormone imbalance.

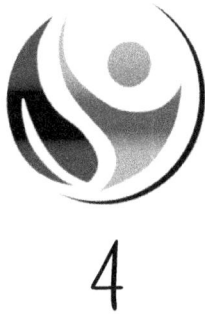

4

Hormonal Health

Do you actually know what hormones do within your body? They are messengers. They send complex messages throughout your body. They are chemicals that work with the central nervous system to send out operating instructions throughout your body. Your hormones are produced by several different glands throughout your body and then put into the bloodstream to send messages where needed. These glands include:

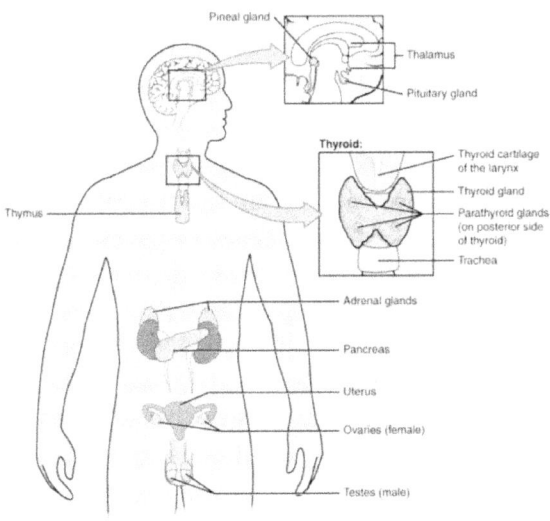

- The Hypothalamus

- The Pituitary Gland

- The Pineal Gland

- The Thyroid

- The Parathyroid

- The Adrenal Gland

- The Ovaries in Women and the Testes in Men

Every time your body goes through a process, hormones tell it when to start and end and everything it should do in between. For example, you go through menstruation because your hormones tell your body to do this.

Different women have different sensitivities to hormones as well. To understand this better, try a little experiment.

Go get a very soft shirt from your closet. Now, run that shirt through your fingers. Feel the fabric. Really experience it with your fingertips. Now, use your knee to feel the fabric. Try to experience it in the same way. You cannot. That's because you have more nerve endings in your fingertips than you have on other parts of your body. Your fingers are made to ensure you can feel and experience.

Your hormones and the receptors throughout your body act in very much the same way. Different organs in your body will be much more sensitive to hormones than others. That means a very small amount of the chemicals can make a very big difference.

Regulation of Your Cycle

I have never had a regular period. I would always hear other girls talking about how they knew exactly which day they would start on and I was amazed. I had no idea that things for me were abnormal. Yes, my period would sometimes start at day 28, but then again, sometimes it would start at day 25 or day 32. Usually, it was late and I have to admit, that resulted in more than one pregnancy scare in my younger years.

No one told me my irregular period was nothing more than a frustration, until I finally mentioned it to a nurse friend in passing. She said I should talk to my doctor and I did. That's when my OBGYN started talking about my hypothalamus. I hate to admit it, but I didn't know what a hypothalamus was or that I even had one. It turns out, mine wasn't working completely right and my hormones were out of balance because of it.

Several different processes go on in your body to ensure you have your menstrual cycle. You may be surprised to know what is actually happening.

Let's talk about the hypothalamus. It is located in your brain and its job is to release hormones. It receives information and then sends out the right signals to properly regulate the body. The hypothalamus monitors how much estrogen and progesterone is being released by your ovaries and then it reacts accordingly. When it is time for the cycle to start, the hypothalamus sends signals to the pituitary gland, also in the brain, and tells it what to do. The pituitary gland then sends out one of two different hormones depending on the time of the month:

- FSH – This is the follicle stimulating hormone and it tells the ovary to create a follicle and it will be able to produce a mature egg.

- LH – This is the luteinizing hormone and it essentially tells the ovary it is time to release the mature egg.

That's just the basics, too. We will get into more detail about the vast network of hormones and messages that create your body.

Here's one thing to note though: hormone levels change every single day. This means they are very hard to pin down with just one blood test. In other words, if you have a hormonal imbalance that is causing you problems, it may not be noticeable in the beginning. The body works on the very premise that hormones are constantly changing, sending messages, and getting stronger or weaker.

Types of Hormones

Now, let's get into a few specific types of hormones in your body that have a direct effect on your sexual health. It's important to understand more about these hormones since it's likely you may not know how they work and regulate your menstrual cycle and sexual health.

Estrogen

You probably have heard the most about estrogen, because it is the most well-known female hormone. It's talked about a lot when referring to women, their sexuality, their fertility, and other changes in their lives. Estrogen is produced by the ovaries and adrenal glands, and is responsible for several important things in your body:

- Because it circulates through the blood stream, it affects the reproductive organs, but it also has an effect on the brain, heart. Liver, bones, and other areas of the body.

- Estrogen tells the uterus to begin creating the lining, (endometrium) so that it will be prepared to support a fertilized egg.

- The hormone controls the changes your body went through during puberty, including growing breasts. '

- During certain times of your life including adolescenthood and then pregnancy, estrogen will regulate metabolic processes, including bone growth and regulation of cholesterol levels.

- Estrogen ensures the vagina and vaginal opening are elastic and strong.

- It helps to prevent loss of bone density in aging women and helps regulate bone growth in adolescent girls.

Essentially, estrogen interacts with almost every single cell you have in your body. It controls a vast network of messages that don't just affect your sexual health, but your overall body health as well.

Androgens

Many people are confused about androgens, which include testosterone, because they refer to these hormones as distinctly male. However, women need androgens too.

They play an important role in fetal development when a woman is pregnant and they certainly have a big role in sexual health and response. Some of the many functions that androgens regulate include:

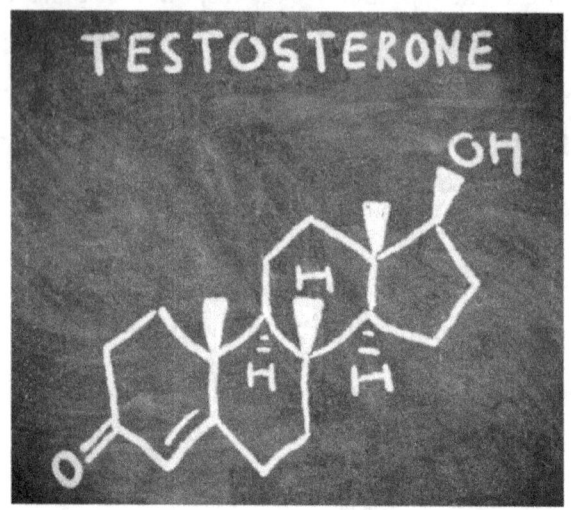

- Growth of body hair during puberty

- Regulation of kidney, liver, and muscle function

- Regulation and health of the reproductive tract (vagina)

- Prevention of bone loss during aging

- Strengthening of sexual desire as well as sexual satisfaction

- Regulation of body functions throughout menopause and afterward

Androgens may often be called "the male hormone", but women have them too, produced by their kidneys and ovaries. They are important and we will even talk about them more later.

Progesterone

The next type of hormone we need to discuss is progesterone. This hormone is specifically connected with pregnancy. It is released in the body, all the time through the ovaries and adrenal glands, but the amount jumps significantly during pregnancy.

This hormone makes sure the uterine lining is mature and prepared to support the fertilized egg. Additionally, it helps to avoid any type of uterine contractions, which could actually put the fetus in harm's way. Finally, progesterone is vital to ensuring the body is ready to provide a safe environment for the baby to grow.

> "Normally, a woman experiences about 20-25 mg of progesterone during her cycle. But during pregnancy, the levels increase to 10 times. The body needs the increased amount of progesterone to both prevent the release of other eggs and to foster the growth of breast-milk glands." (Jackson)

Progesterone is one of the easiest hormone measurements used to determine pregnancy. A spike in this hormone points directly to a fertilized egg and implantation.

Thyroid

The thyroid gland produces hormones that regulate many things throughout the body, such as bone growth and weight. It is also connected to sexual health. More and more studies have shown that women who have a low sex drive, also have poor thyroid production.

Women who have hypothyroidism tend to have a lower sex drive. When these women underwent thyroid treatment, they were able to recover their sex drive. So, a malfunction in the thyroid process also has an effect on your sexual health.

Importance of Balance

Now that you understand everything that hormones do in your body, let's stop a minute and consider why balanced hormones are so important. Long-term imbalance of hormones has been connected to a variety of conditions, and we will talk about those next. For now, though, it's important to consider the need for a proactive approach.

There are many different things that could completely throw your hormone balance out of whack, so to speak. Sometimes, women experience an imbalance after pregnancy, after puberty, when they are stressed, or during menopause. Some women simply have a hormone imbalance for no noticeable reason. In any case, these imbalances can make you and your body very unhappy, and for various reasons, your body may not be able to get things straightened out on its own.

That's why hormone treatments have become so popular. More and more women are understanding just how important it is to have hormone balance. They are seeking methods to actually get things straight in droves, so that they can be healthier sexually happier in their lives.

> "Hormone fluctuations can take a strong body and render it weak, unpredictable, and unreliable. However, hormonal problems should not be seen as an inevitable part of being a woman or something that we should just accept. Hormonal problems that occur at different stages of life do not have to be accepted as normal." (It's All about Balance)

Hormone balance can be achieved through many different treatments, along with changes in your life. We will discuss those in further detail in the next chapter.

Symptoms of Imbalance

My name is Kaly and I am only 30 years old. That's why it came as a total surprise to me when one of my friends suggested something might be wrong with my hormones. I thought those kinds of problems only happened for women in menopause or women who had babies. I am single, childless and years away from menopause I hope. But, there were things going on.

To start with, I have been overweight for a long time. I am not obese by any means, but I am very curvy. I have tried numerous different diets, exercise programs, and weight loss methods. None of them worked. I mean, I could drop a pound or two here and there, but it made no real difference.

When my friend was talking about her own struggles with hormone imbalance, she started naming things, and I thought "oh my gosh! I had no idea those things had anything to do with my weight problems." You see, I was experiencing fingernails that broke easily and didn't grow well, hair that just looked…well dead, I had very little energy, and my skin really could have looked better.

It turns out, as she told me, that all of these things were linked together – hormones. So, I made an appointment at the doctor's office. I soon found out that yes, I had a hormone imbalance all due to hypothyroidism. My thyroid wasn't working correctly and was not producing the hormones my body needed. This explained everything, my doctor told me, and then she started me on replacement therapy. It has changed my life!"

Unfortunately, many women think that the only time they could suffer from hormonal imbalance is during menopause, but that isn't always true. In fact, the imbalance issues can affect any woman, at any age, for a wide variety of reasons.

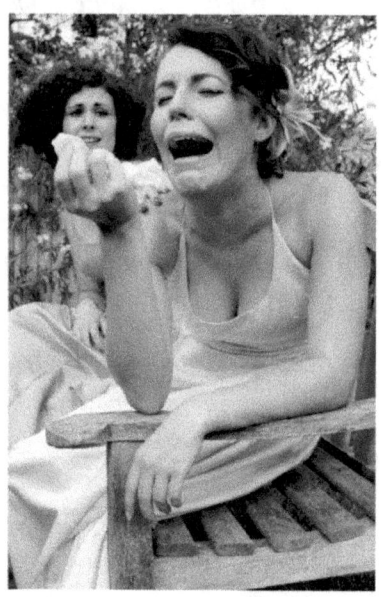

Symptoms List

Let's go through the list of symptoms associated with hormonal imbalance in women. We will break those symptoms down into several different categories, including imbalances in certain types of hormones, as well as general imbalance.

General

There are quite a few different symptoms that can be connected, to a hormone imbalance. Of course, many of them could point to other conditions too, so it is important to discuss your symptoms with a physician:

Menstrual Changes (Irregular Period)	Lack of Sex Drive or Low Libido
Uncontrollable Acne or Adult Acne	Regular Headaches
Oily Skin or Very Dry Skin	Weight Gain Despite Dieting and
Hair Growth on Unexpected Body Parts	Endometriosis
Constant Fatigue Even with Rest	Irregular Water Retention
Feelings of Dizziness	PMS or PMDD
Generalized Anxiety with no Identifiable	Regular or Recurrent Urinary Tract

Now, let's talk about symptoms or conditions associated with specific types of hormonal imbalances.

Estrogen

High Estrogen

PMS	Mood Swings
Migraine Headaches	Insomnia
Severe Cramps	Skin Conditions
Fibroids in the Uterus	Sore or Enlarged Breasts
Depression	Miscarriage
Weight Gain	Excessive Facial Hair
Hot Flashes	Loss of Hair
Irregular Menstruation	Low Sex Drive
Memory Loss and Foggy Thinking	

Low Estrogen

Fatigue	Loss of Sex Drive
Night Sweats and Hot Flashes	Memory Problems
Vaginal Dryness	Difficulty with Concentration
Dry Skin	Atherosclerosis
Panic Attacks	Joint Pain
Depression	Recurrent Vaginal Infections
Anxiety	Unexplained Low Self Esteem
Headaches	

Low estrogen levels are most often associated with menopause, but there are other causes, including illness and some medical treatments. Women who are overweight and have high blood pressure are more prone to high levels of estrogen.

Progesterone

High Progesterone

Breast Tenderness and Swelling	Recurrent Yeast Infections
Mood Swings	Dizziness
Sleepiness	Feeling Bloated

Low Progesterone

Depression	Low Blood Sugar
Fibrous Cysts in Breasts	Water Retention
Unexplained Weight Gain	Panic Attacks
Irregular Periods	Heavy Menstruation
Vaginal Dryness	

Excess estrogen and problems with insulin can lead to low levels of progesterone. High progesterone can be caused by a number of different factors, such as birth control pills.

Androgens

High Androgens

Excess Acne	Obesity
Hair Growth on Face and Chin	Infertility
Thin Hair on the Head	Irregular Periods
Polycystic Ovaries	
High Cholesterol	

Low Androgens

Low Sex Drive	Fatigue
Vaginal Dryness	

High Androgen levels can actually have serious consequences on your health, when left untreated. They can lead to diabetes, high blood pressure, high cholesterol, and heart disease. Low androgens have also been connected to health conditions, such as bone loss.

Overall, when hormone imbalances of any type are left untreated, they can lead to a number of different serious conditions beyond just feeling "off". They can include:

Infertility and Miscarriage Uterine Cysts

Infertility and Miscarriage	Uterine Cysts
Osteoporosis	Heart Disease
Ovarian Cysts	Breast Cancer
Endometriosis	Mood Disorders

That's why it is so important to treat hormone imbalances when they are discovered!

The Imbalance Quiz

Here is a simple quiz you can use to determine if you may have a hormone imbalance. Below, you will be introduced to six different symptom groups. Check off any of the symptoms you experience. If you experience more than two symptoms in any one category, then you may have an imbalance in that area. Additionally, if you check off numerous symptoms in several categories, it is likely you may have an imbalance.

Category 1:

Premenstrual Syndrome	Infertility
Weight Gain for no Reason	Early Miscarriage
Insomnia	Anxiety
Painful Breasts	Headaches along with Your Cycle

Category 2:

Vaginal Dryness	Pain during Sex
Night Sweats or Hot Flashes	Frequent Bladder Infections
Depression	Lethargy

Category 3:

Bloating	Crying for no Reason
Weight Gain	Heavy Menstruation
Anxiety	Migraines
Insomnia	Gallbladder Issues
Flushed Face	Tenderness in the Breast
Cervical Dysplasia	Mood Swings

Category 4:

The same symptoms as category 1 and 3.

Those symptoms could also point to a condition called estrogen dominance and a lack of progesterone.

Category 5:

Excess Acne	Pain in the Middle of the Cycle
Facial Hair	Polycystic Ovaries
Ovarian Cysts	Blood Sugar Problems
Infertility	Thinning Hair

Category 6:

Extreme Fatigue	Inability to Think Clearly
Dry Skin	Discolored Spots on the Face
Blood Sugar Problems	Low Blood Pressure
Inability to Exercise	

These symptoms could refer to a lack of cortisol, a hormone created in the adrenal glands.

Why Imbalance Happens

There are quite a few reasons why hormone imbalances occur and they can affect women of different ages. Let's explore more of the possible ways hormone imbalance may occur.

Adrenal Exhaustion

I never knew that the adrenal glands could get tired. Turns out they can. So, when I talked to my doctor because tired all the time and very moody, she suggested that they do some blood work.

Then, she started asking me how often I spent time stressed out. I told her that I did have an extremely stressful job. I had no idea that my chronic stress could actually cause things to go wrong. It turns out my glands were exhausted, as she put it, and this was messing with my hormones.

————————

Your adrenal glands contribute to several different types of hormones and are very important for estrogen and progesterone function. They also create cortisol whenever you are in stressful or frightening situations. If the adrenal glands are no longer working properly, this can lead to a variety of hormone disturbances.

Eating Disorders

"I struggled with an eating disorder for many years and I didn't really realize what was going wrong with my body. I thought that the Anorexia would actually mess with my hormones. I didn't know that I was actually harming myself to that extent."

When I started to get help with my disorder, I also started talking to a medical doctor. She asked me if my periods were regular. I had to admit that I had not had a period in five months. She explained to me what was happening in my body and she explained how the eating disorder was causing my hormonal imbalances. It's no wonder I felt exhausted all of the time. I am proud to say that I did get my life in order and through counseling, I was able to overcome the disorder, and I have gotten my hormones back in balance.

Eating disorders like anorexia and bulimia can actually cause hormone imbalances. When the body is going through the stress, caused by these disorders, it generally stops producing important reproductive hormones and often leads to women having irregular or absent periods.

PCOS

When I was about 24, I noticed that I was having trouble with…well…there's no other way to explain it than I had a moustache. It was so embarrassing! I tried bleaching it for a while, but then switched to waxing. I had no idea that this problem was actually a symptom of a hormonal imbalance, as well as a condition called PCOS.

When my husband and I tried to get pregnant with no luck, we went to a fertility specialist who discovered the problem.

Polycystic ovarian syndrome is caused by a hormone condition and it causes additional hormonal imbalances. It is created from high levels of androgens and can lead to high levels of luteinizing hormones and low FSH.

Post-Partum

I thought that having a baby would be a completely joyous, happy event. I thought I would be excited and happy every single moment. Then, in the days after my little boy was born, I didn't understand what was going on with my body. I was depressed. I was tired all the time. I couldn't stop crying. I even resented the baby. I hate admitting that. I thought I must be a horrible mother.

Then, someone told me that post-partum can come along with serious hormonal imbalances that can even result in post-partum depression. It was only then that I sought help from my doctor.

After having a baby, some women are at risk for hormonal imbalances. For example, the thyroid can begin to malfunction, by either becoming over or under active.

Birth Control Pills

I took birth control pills for a decade. I didn't want to get pregnant, so I started them when I was in college. I did not stop until my early 30s when my husband and I wanted to have a baby. I was a little surprised at what happened when I stopped the pill.

The only way to put it is things went crazy. Well, I felt like I went crazy. I was tired, irritable, moody, and I would cry for no reason at all. I couldn't get control of my emotions. It was a very difficult time. When I talked to my doctor, I learned that, because I was on birth control pills for so long, my body had to readjust to the hormonal changes and this threw everything out of balance.

Because birth control pills regulate hormone production, they can, at times, lead to hormonal imbalances, including low testosterone and androgens. This happens most commonly when a woman has been taking birth control pills for a very long time. However, when taking birth control pills, they can actually help to regulate hormones since they keep everything even, throughout the month. It's important to talk to your doctor to determine if birth control pills will be the right option for you. If you have been on the pill for a long time and you are getting ready to stop, you should discuss any hormone imbalance concerns you have with your physician.

Menopause

It was that dreaded time. I was 50 when it started happening. The hot flashes. The night sweats. The irritability. It all began for me. I was going through menopause. I chalked it all up to normal. It's a part of life, right? Then, things started to get rough when I didn't even feel like being intimate with my husband. I was very dry down there and it seemed like I was just, well, getting old.

I had no idea there were ways to treat this and that through hormone supplements, I could get my life back.

Obviously, menopause leads to hormonal imbalances, since the ovaries begin to stop making the reproductive hormones needed. Additionally, there is a condition called premature menopause, when the ovaries begin to fail at an early age. Premature menopause is not common, but it does happen. In any case, menopause is the most common reason why women experience hormone imbalances.

Stress

I have a high stress job and I have a high stress home life. My work as a paramedic means I am responsible for saving people when they are sick or injured. It's stressful and I probably add to the stress level by expecting so much out of myself. Then, I get home, and as much as I love my son, his autism adds to my stress levels. It's a lot of work and it is a lot of stress.

I had no idea that my body was actually continuously producing hormones to keep the stress in check. I also didn't know that this would eventually mess my hormone levels up. I didn't know all of this until my doctor announced to me that my adrenal glands were exhausted.

When your body is under stress for too long of a time, your hormone producing glands cannot keep up. They will continually be producing hormones designed to deal with stress and this causes disruptions in the natural hormone process. This can lead to a wide variety of imbalance problems, that affect your sex life as well as your everyday health.

Environmental Chemicals

I live out in the country, right in the middle of several farms. It's the same place I have lived all of my life and where my parents have lived too. I knew that pesticides aren't exactly safe for people, but I didn't know they actually had the ability to damage my hormones. I found out from my doctor that my body actually thought it had more hormones than it did, because the pesticides were actually confusing it.

It is believed that certain chemicals found in the environment, like pesticides and hormones used in foods, can actually mimic estrogen in the human body. As a result, your body may stop making estrogen, believing there is enough and this could lead to a deficiency.

It's obvious that an imbalance in hormones can have a variety of side effects on your body, including on your sexual health. People often don't really realize how much hormones have an effect on their wellbeing. Instead, they often see hormones as nothing more than something to blame their bad moods on. The reality is that hormones play a dramatic role in your overall health, your sexual health, and your daily life. That's why it is so important that you consider treatment options when you and your doctor determine that you have an imbalance.

In the next chapter, let's discuss treatments available to get your hormones back in order. There are numerous different options available depending on which hormone is out of balance and your current situation. You may just be surprised to find out what is available to you to address your sexual and general health issues.

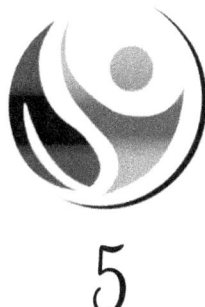

5

Hormone Imbalance Treatment Options

Once I found out that I had a hormonal imbalance, I thought there would be nothing to change my situation. I assumed that I would just have to live with the problems for the rest of my life. Then, my doctor presented me with several different treatment options. That certainly was a surprise to me.

*Not only was there something that could be done, but there were actually **several** things that could be done. After discussing my options with my physician, we determined that I should take bioidentical hormone supplements. My doctor recommended these, because they come so close to replicating the hormones in my body.*

When things started to straighten out for me, I was glad that I found out there were treatments that could help.

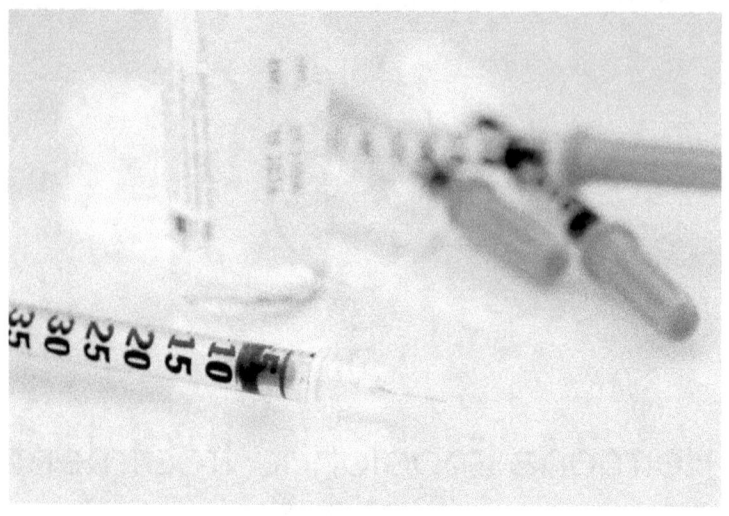

There really are a number of different treatments available for hormonal imbalance. Some of them use traditional methods that are considered "tried and true". Others use the most cutting edge technology and research to offer more finely tuned treatments. In this chapter, we will discuss everything from what's considered the conventional treatments to the newest options available.

Depending on your body and the type of imbalance you have, it will be important to find the right treatment, for the best results.

Conventional Treatment Options

Medications

We will start with the most common category of hormone treatments: different types of medications. Medications for hormone imbalances have been in use for a very long time. However, even they have changed with newer and better technology. So, be sure to consider all types of medications and determine with your doctor, what will work the best for you and your health needs.

Pills, Creams, and Injections

There are actually different types of hormones that can be used to treat imbalances. Called bioidentical hormone therapy (BHT), these treatments use hormone replacements that closely mirror the hormones already in your body, for the best results. Pills, injections and creams have been the most common options for hormone therapy. Here are some of the reasons certain types of treatments may not be all that effective:

- The pills are made from a gelatin capsule that are not easily absorbed by the body.

- Creams are placed on the skin of the stomach or the inner thighs and are absorbed into the body. Absorption is questionable due to placement, time of day and consistent use.

- Injections are available specifically for testosterone treatments when women need a low dose testosterone supplement. You learn how to give yourself the injections, however, injections can spike the level of testosterone and can cause the body to stop producing testosterone naturally.

Some of the most common (not BHRT) medications in this category include:

Estrace (Pill)	Estrasorb (Cream)
Estrace (Cream)	Prometrium (Pill)
Alora (Patch)	Combipatch (Patch)
Estrogel (Gel)	Prefest (Pill)
Evamist (Spray)	Climera Pro (Patch)
Vagifem (Pill)	

Pellet Therapy

Another option for bio-identical hormone treatment is pellet therapy. This therapy involves a doctor injecting the medication in pellet form, underneath the skin. The pellets then react when the body is in need of hormones and releases them as needed.

Did you know that hormone replacement using pellet implants has been around for more than 70 years? In fact, scientists have published positive research on the benefits of this therapy in authoritative international journals, for decades.

Bio-identical pellet therapy was originally developed in Europe during the 1930s. It proved an excellent treatment for hormone deficiencies, especially during menopause. The highly-respected pioneer of endocrinology, Dr. Robert B. Greenblatt, learned about this method and introduced it to his U.S. colleagues in 1939. Today, practitioners on five continents use pellet implants to restore hormonal balance in men and women of all ages.

PELLET IMPLANTS: SAFE, EFFECTIVE, CONVENIENT BHRT

When properly administered, the pellet delivery system provides safe and effective BHRT. In fact, it remains the only form of delivery that closely mirrors what the human ovary and testicle do. This method ensures the same steady, around-the-clock, low dosages the body once created. You won't have to change patches, rub on creams, or remember to take a pill. Pellet implants deliver more when the body needs it—like during exercise or periods of stress.

BENEFITS OF BIOIDENTICAL PELLETS:

The only method that allows the body to control the release of hormone—raising levels

when more is needed and decreasing it when requiring less.

Deliver a very low dosage continuously, 24/7.

Releases testosterone and/or estradiol directly into the bloodstream, bypassing the gastrointestinal system and liver.

Consistently proven more effective than oral, injected, or topical methods with regard to sexual function, mood and cognitive function, metabolic function, bone density, urinary and vaginal problems, lipid profiles, breast health and hormone ratios.

Typically last from 3 to 6 months.

Conjugated Equine Estrogens

Another type of hormone replacement medications come from hormones extracted from a pregnant horse's urine. This medication, called Premarin, mimics the human hormones. There are some concerns about this choice of medication since these hormones tend to have numerous side effects and the humane treatment of animals is a concern for some women.

Synthetic Hormones

These hormone medications are made in a laboratory and do not have any natural substances in them. As a result, they can to have some adverse effects on a woman's body.

When you begin considering your options for hormone treatments, one thing you will notice right away is that there are two major categories: bioidentical and synthetic. It's important that you understand both of these and know which is best for your own needs.

Bio-Identical vs. Synthetic Hormones

When I first started taking hormone supplements, bioidentical hormones were unheard of, or they were unheard of to me. I was presented with only one option: a synthetic hormone created in a laboratory, My doctor explained that there were quite a few different side effects that I could expect and sure enough, I dealt with a lot of them. It wasn't fun. But, what other choice did I have? My body wasn't producing hormones correctly because I was going through the early stages before menopause. I thought I had to take the meds.

Then, when I had to start seeing a new doctor because my husband and I relocated, the physician asked if I had ever considered taking bioidentical hormones. I had never heard of them before, but once he started explaining them, I knew it was the right decision for me. Since I started taking these medications, my hormones have been much more in balance and I haven't had to deal with any of those nasty side effects.

Synthetic hormones are created in a laboratory by a pharmaceutical company. This means they will have a patented formula that is the same for every single patient who takes them. The only thing that will be different is the actual number of milligrams that the patient takes. These synthetic hormones are not the same as human hormones and they do a poor job of mimicking the endogenous hormones in your body. Here is a rundown of the problems of synthetic hormones:

• They are not tailored to each person's body.

• They do not mimic natural hormones.

• They come along with a wide variety of side effects.

Bioidentical hormones are quite different, because they use natural materials to mimic the endogenous hormones already in the patient's body. Because they are an exact replica structurally, they integrate more naturally in the body and they have little or no side effects. Bioidentical hormones are made from a few different plant sources such as soy and wild yams. They are not completely created in a laboratory.

So, what does that mean for your body? BHRT, or bioidentical hormone replacement therapy, is considered much safer and much more effective at treating hormone imbalances.

I Am a Woman –– Why Are We Talking about Testosterone?

Several times throughout this chapter and previously in the book, we have mentioned testosterone (one of the androgens). You may have been scratching your head, thinking "ok, that makes no sense! I am a woman, why on earth would I need testosterone?" After all, this is considered the male hormone, right? Most people associate testosterone with manliness, muscles, and other distinctly masculine features. That's why it certainly may come as a surprise to them, when they learn women need testosterone, too!

Your adrenal glands and ovaries both make a small amount of testosterone. It's not nearly the amount found in a man's body, but it is present and it is needed. Testosterone levels in women are linked to one very important thing: the sex drive. So, when women have low t-levels, they may lose their libido.

When a woman is about 20 years old, her testosterone levels and production peaks. Then, it begins to taper off with age, and that can affect sex drive. There are other cases in which the testosterone levels may drop dramatically, such as:

- Total hysterectomy in which the patient must have their ovaries removed,

- Having a condition in which the patient's adrenal system is not working properly, or

- Women who take medications that may interrupt testosterone production.

Testosterone Therapy

When I told my doctor that my sex drive was really low (that was a fun conversation. I had to psyche myself up in advance. "Jamie, you can do this!" I told myself over and over again), she told me that I might need testosterone therapy. I was so confused. I am a woman, why on this earth would I need testosterone?

I quickly learned that even women have testosterone and it is directly tied to the libido. Well, I certainly learned something new! Once my doctor started me on a low does testosterone therapy, my sex drive has improved. My husband and I are very happy with those results.

While considering a new treatment option, low dose testosterone therapy in women has shown to be very promising. Testosterone pellet threapy is designed to replace the lost testosterone needed in a woman's body, so that they may continue to enjoy a healthy sex drive.

There are cases in which testosterone therapy is not a healthy option, including:

- Women who are or may be pregnant, since the testosterone can affect the unborn baby

- Women who have or have had breast or uterine cancer

- Women who have been diagnosed with heart disease or high cholesterol

- Women who have or have had liver disease

Generally, testosterone therapy was used solely in women who have gone through menopause, but Doctors today also treat younger women suffering from with low sex drive.

Testosterone is not just a hormone for men, even though it is more prevalent in the male body. However, it is an important hormone in your chemical makeup. You need testosterone, because it has a direct effect on your libido. To maintain a healthy sex drive, you need a certain amount of testosterone in your body.

New and Better Treatment Options

Once upon a time, the only hormone therapy treatment options came in the form of synthetic pills or creams created in a laboratory. This wasn't the best option because many women experienced negative side effects and they didn't get much relief from the therapy. Then came Premarin, the more natural hormone therapy made from pregnant mare's urine. However, this still didn't fully integrate into a woman's body and that meant it wasn't as effective as needed.

That's why the very best treatment option is also the newest: bioidentical hormone replacement therapy or BHRT. As mentioned earlier, this option perfectly mimics the hormones in your body, so that the medications integrate well, with no side effects and better results.

Bioidentical hormones are still relatively new, and they have been a source of debate ever since they were allowed on the market. Some people do not believe they could work. However, the research shows that this type of hormone replacement will have the best results of integrating into the body. Obviously, if the hormones mimic those in your body, they are going to do a much better job or replacement and treatment, for symptoms related to hormonal imbalances.

Even if you are already on hormone balance medications, it may be a very good idea to consider other options. Medication has changed drastically in the past few years. Now there are hormone replacement therapies that closely mirror the hormones in your own body. So, if you are already on prescriptions, go ahead and discuss with your doctor to see if you have other options. There may be a better medication to consider, if you have been taking something considered older or outdated.

We have talked about your body, your sexual health, and hormones. You likely have learned a lot about how you actually work, but what if things still aren't right down there? Let's talk about this problem and the various solutions you could consider in the next chapter.

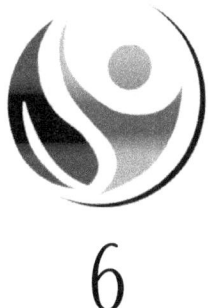

6

I'm Just Not Working down There Anymore

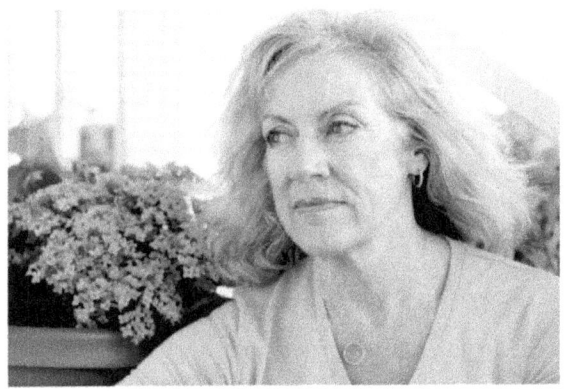

After reading all of this information so far, what's going through your mind? It may be something like:

> "It's all well and good. Yes, hormones. Yes, replacement. But, that doesn't change my problem. I am just not working *down there* anymore. Am I supposed to just live with this?"

The answer to your question is most certainly not! If you are experiencing one of the many issues that can result in painful sex or loss of sex drive, and you have been suffering in silence, it is important for things to change. This is not how you should live, no matter your age and no matter if you have gone through menopause or not.

There are, unfortunately, a lot of different things that can go wrong down there for women, like vaginal dryness, incontinence, loss of sensation, inability to orgasm, and loss of sex drive. It's all very frustrating, but the good news is that there are ways to treat all of it.

The Whys

"There are changes in the female sexual response cycle, as women age, that affect their reaction to sexual intimacy. Libido is maintained until quite late in the aging process. With aging, there is delayed or diminished vaginal lubrication, vasocongestion, diminished frequency of contraction of the vagina, and decreased frequency of orgasm." (Kuzmarov, 2008)

Doctors don't fully understand all of the whys related this decline, but they do know it is largely related to hormones. As your body ages, it stops making the same amount of estrogen, progesterone, and androgens. As a result, sex drive begins to decrease and sexual dysfunctions begin to arise. Some of these problems and the whys that they happen include:

- Vaginal dryness occurs as estrogen levels lower. This leads to discomfort during intercourse.

- Vasocongestion leads to less blood flow to the sexual and reproductive organs. This makes it harder to climax and to enjoy sexual arousal.

- The vagina doesn't have the same elasticity as it did as estrogen levels decline and this leads to less feeling during intercourse.

- The urethra begins to widen and change form as hormone levels change, and this leads to more incontinence problems.

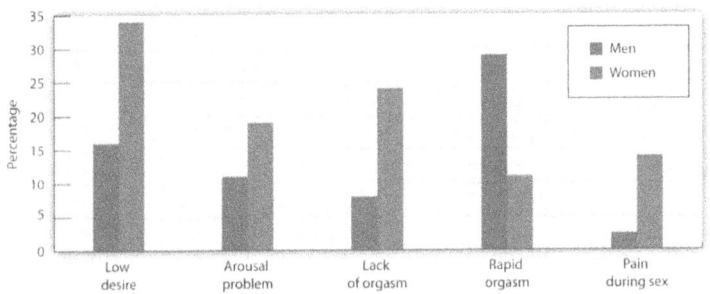

The above chart, provided by <u>Flatworld Knowledge</u>, shows the drastic difference in sexual dysfunction in men and women. As you can see from the chart, women are much more likely to suffer loss of sexual desire, lack of arousal, inability to orgasm, and pain during intercourse itself.

Now, let's talk about some various conditions and treatments specifically.

Vaginal Dryness

Ever since I turned 45, I have been running into a big problem. I am dry down there all the time and that includes when I am turned on. It doesn't just cause problems during sex either. It feels sore and even swollen sometimes. It is absolutely miserable!

And when it comes to the sex with my husband...well...let's just say it isn't fun anymore. That doesn't mean I don't want it. I do. I enjoy sex as much as the next woman, but it is very hard to enjoy it when things hurt. The burning is just too much and the only alternative we have found so far is to load up on lube. Is there any other solution for vaginal dryness?

Vaginal dryness is often one of the first symptoms associated with female aging, Estrogen is the hormone responsible for ensuring the vagina can lubricate itself, and as the hormone is available in lower amounts, things dry out. Symptoms of vaginal dryness include:

Burning, especially during intercourse	The feeling of urgency for urination
Soreness	Urinary tract infections
Bleeding after intercourse	Itching around the vaginal opening

Although the main cause of vaginal dryness is menopause, which is likely the culprit in the story at the beginning of the section, it is not the only cause. In fact, even younger women can experience this condition. Essentially, anything that can cause estrogen levels to drop within the body can cause vaginal dryness. These can include:

Childbirth	Sjogren's Syndrome
Breast Feeding a Baby	Allergy Medications
Surgical Ovary Removal	Cold Medications
Certain Immune Disorders	Breast Cancer Medications
Cancer Therapy on or near the Ovaries	Too Much Douching
Cigarette Smoking	

While hormone replacement therapy can treat vaginal dryness in many cases, it is not always going to be a complete solution. There are other things you can do to relieve the pain and discomfort associated with this condition. We will discuss these next.

Lubricate and Moisturize

Because the vagina does become dry, you will need to consider the use of lubricants and moisturizers. You have options that are easy to obtain, since they are available in almost any drugstore or even in pharmacy sections of super stores, like Wal-Mart. When you choose vaginal lubricants, make sure to avoid oil based types if you use condoms during sexual intercourse. The oil based lubricants will break down the material of the condom.

Some of the most popular lubricants available in almost any pharmacy include:

Liquid Silk (lubricant)	Replens (vaginal moisturizer)
Astroglide (lubricant)	Carrageenan (lubricant)
Oh! (lubricant)	K-Y Brand Products (lubricant)

Another way of treating vaginal dryness, through extra lubrication, is available in the form of localized estrogen treatments. There are creams and other ways to offer a healthier vagina overall. A few of these options include:

- Vagifem, which is a suppository that is placed in the vagina to provide estrogen in the local area only.

- Estring, which is a flexible ring that releases estrogen and is placed inside the vagina next to the cervix.

- Estradoil, which is a cream that can be applied to the vagina and vulva area.

Nutrition

Now, let's talk about some changes you can make to your diet that can also help with vaginal dryness. Some of these foods will actually help the condition, while others will help you maintain overall vaginal health. Of course, the healthier your vagina is, the better it will feel. The foods you should consider eating include the following:

Probiotics

Yogurt	Miso
Kimchi	Kefir
Sauerkraut	

Infection Fighters

Cranberry Juice	Cutting back on alcohol and caffeine

Foods that Help with Moisture

Water	Olive Oil
Avocados	Wheat Germ
Seeds	Fruits and Veggies
Nuts	

Vaginal dryness doesn't have to be "just a part of life". In fact, it doesn't have to be a problem at all. Depending on the specific causes of the dryness for you, you can use a selection of different treatments to make your life more comfortable.

Whether you choose creams and lubricants, topical estrogen, changes in diet, or stretching exercises, you will find they will ensure more comfort for you. Sexual intercourse is a healthy part of your life and your relationships, and it shouldn't be avoided just because you are experiencing the dryness. By using treatments and making changes, you can enjoy comfort and pleasure during sex. Remember that sex should not be painful and vaginal dryness is a common cause of this type of pain. Be sure to consider your options instead, of just dealing with the discomfort.

These treatments provide the needed estrogen to the area so that your vagina will be stimulated and will begin creating its natural lubricant as it used to. These localized estrogen products are only available by prescription so you would need to discuss your concerns with your physician.

Stretching

Often, women who experience vaginal dryness also deal with pain during intercourse because the muscles in the vaginal wall are no longer as resilient as they used to be. As the muscles become more rigid, they do not allow as much stretching which leads to discomfort.

To help this, you can do stretching exercises. This will help to minimize the pain when you are engaging in penetrative intercourse. Your vaginal health is important, even if you don't believe you will be involved in sex anytime soon. Doing these exercises can help for a variety of different reasons. Let's talk about two different things you can do for vaginal stretching.

• Kegel Exercises

The first thing you need to do is locate your pelvic floor muscles. These are the muscles that will actually stop urination, so the easiest way to find them is when you have to go to the bathroom. Once you know where your pelvic floor muscles are and how to control them, do the following:

Lie down on your back and tighten the muscles, holding them tight for five seconds. Then release them for five seconds. Then repeat this exercise five times in a row. Work your way up slowly to being able to hold the muscle contraction for 10 seconds at a time.

Make sure when you work on this, you do not hold your breath or tighten your buttocks.

If you do this three times a day, you will find this does a good job of toning up your vaginal muscles. Kegels can also help with minor urinary leakage too.

• Stretching

If you have trouble with your vagina not stretching enough during intercourse and causing pain, then this stretching method will help.

When you are in the shower or bathtub, make sure your fingers are wet and then insert one or two of them in your vagina. Begin making a circular motion with your fingers, slowly pushing against all of the walls of your vagina. Then, put your index finger close to the vaginal opening and begin pressing gently outward in all directions.

When you do this on a daily basis, your vagina will begin to respond and become more elastic during sexual intercourse. Make yourself a reminder note you see in the shower, so that you will not forget to do the stretches. Some women choose to write on their shampoo or body wash bottle with a marker. Anything you do to help you remember will help and this will give you better results, so you can have a more pain-free sex life.

Loss of Sensation

I had my little girl five years ago. I gave birth to her naturally, which is a fact I am proud of, but I have to admit that things haven't been the same down there ever since. It's not really what I expected too. I have lost sensation. I just don't feel stimulation like I used to and this makes it very, very hard for me to have an orgasm.

And that fact puts a damper on our sex lives. We engage in sex and then I don't climax, so the questions arise:

"Amber, am I doing something wrong?" or "Am I just not good anymore?" These are the kinds of questions my husband would ask.

I kept trying to explain to him that it hadn't anything to do with his abilities. It was me. But, my husband has a bit of that stereotypical male ego and he was convinced I wasn't attracted to him anymore. We virtually stopped having sex.

It was a nightmare.

Then, I found out about the O-Shot®."

The O-Shot® has been featured on Dr. Oz, ABC's Good Morning America.

Amber, like many other women, began to lose sensitivity and sensation in her vaginal area after childbirth. It happens often, but it isn't the only cause. Women can lose sensitivity as they approach menopause or for other reasons and medical conditions.

One of the newest methods to treat this sensation loss is called the O-Shot®.

> "Up to 25% of women have an orgasmic dysfunction, which is defined as the persistent or recurrent delay or absence of orgasm following a normal sexual excitement phase. The list of reasons this might happen is long and includes medications, hormone issues, medical problems, or relationship issues." (Streicher, 2014)

Since lack of sensation and inability to orgasm is a problem for many women, the O-Shot® could be a viable option.

Here are a few statistics that may surprise you. They are listed according to the *International Journal of Pharmaceutical Compounding.*

- Only 25% of women, according to studies, are able to achieve orgasm during intercourse.

- More than 40% of women are not able to achieve sexual satisfaction through clitoral stimulation and orgasm.

- A surprising number of women between ages 18 and 80 do not even know what it feels like to experience orgasm. (Scream Cream)

The O-Shot®

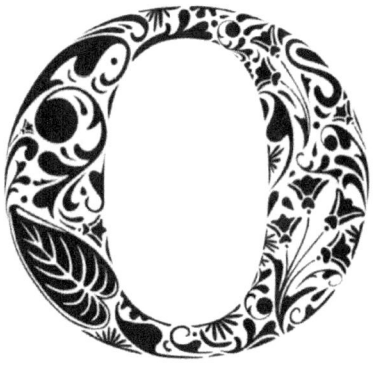

It certainly sounds like some sort of drug. That's what most women would think right away, but it isn't. In fact, the O-Shot® is very natural, because it uses your platelets from your own blood. In the procedure, the platelets are injected into your vaginal tissue, which will attract stem cells to your reproductive area. This is said to create healthier tissue in the whole area for a healthier vagina and more fulfilling sex life.

Patients who have had the O-Shot® have reported improvements in the following ways:

Better vaginal lubrication	More sensation during sex
Greater sensitivity to clitoral stimulation	More frequent orgasms
Decreased pain from intercourse	Stronger orgasms
Tighter vaginal opening	More youthful looking skin around the
Higher sex drive	Help with urinary incontinence

The O-Shot® is a type of treatment referred to as PRP, the same treatment can be used on many different parts of the body.

PRP Treatment

PRP treatment stands for platelet rich plasma. This is a treatment process that uses platelets in the blood plasma

81

from the patient's own bloodstream. Essentially, the platelets can be injected into different tissues to heal and rejuvenate muscles, ligaments, joints, and tendons.

In recent years, doctors have learned that PRP treatment can also be used for vaginal rejuvenation and something called the Vampire FaceLift®, which we will discuss later.

How Does It Work?

PRP treatment works by increasing the number of reparative cells in the area. For example, when the O-Shot® is used in the vaginal tissue, your body will send more stem cells to that area to repair any damage to the tissues. As a result, the reparative cells go to work toward rejuvenation.

Because the O-Shot® uses natural blood platelets from your own body, you don't have to worry about chemical side effects. Instead, it offers benefits that actually go beyond helping women who have trouble achieving orgasm.

Incontinence

"I had always heard the jokes when I was pregnant..."Don't expect to laugh or cough again without peeing!" other mothers would tell me. I laughed it off at the time. Then, after I had my child, I did notice things would get leaky from time to time. It wasn't that bad though. I only experienced it when I laughed really hard, coughed or sneezed really hard, or went running. It was something I could live with.

Then, when I hit age 50, things started going downhill in a hurry. The urinary incontinence has continued to become a worse and worse problem. Now, I have the urge to pee almost all

*the time and there is so much leakiness that I have
to use panty liners every single day.*

It's frustrating!"

Female urinary incontinence is a common in many women, especially as they age or have a baby. The problem can range from a few drops here and there to a serious problem that requires the constant use of incontinence pads.

Causes

The most common type of urinary incontinence in women is called "stress incontinence" and it happens when the pelvic floor muscles stretch and do not return to their normal strength. This often occurs after childbirth or after a serious weight gain. Stress incontinence can be made worse by smoking.

This occurs when the muscles that control and close off the urethra, become worn or tired, rendering them incapable of working properly. Any extra pressure to those muscles like exercise, strenuous activity, laughing, sneezing, and coughing, can cause leakage.

Other causes of incontinence include:

• Urge incontinence due to overactive bladder, bladder irritation, emotional stress, stroke, or Parkinson's disease.

• Total incontinence can be caused by illness, injury, or treatments that completely destroy the pelvic floor muscles.

As a woman ages, the incontinence problem tends to get worse. This has been linked to, of all things, hormonal imbalances.

Treatments

There are different levels of treatment for incontinence. We have already discussed one that has shown to be effective. The O-Shot® was designed for vaginal rejuvenation, but women continue to report that the treatment helps with their incontinence. Here are a few other treatment options:

• Behavior Training

Bladder training is a method used in cases when the woman cannot control her bladder. It has less to do with the pelvic floor muscles and more to do with an overactive bladder, which worsens with age. You will need to create a bathroom diary. This will be a list of every single time you have the urge to go and every time you have a leak.

• Kegel Exercises

We have already discussed kegel exercises as a method to relieve pain from sexual intercourse, so you already know how to go about the training. Kegel exercises will strengthen the pelvic floor muscles overall, and that means they can be helpful for dealing with stress incontinence.

If you do kegel exercises, you need to make sure you do them daily to see results. They will not work if you do them only sporadically.

• Medication

"I never even imagined that there was medication that could be used to help with incontinence. I kind of thought that I would be dealing with my condition for good. When my doctor diagnosed me with stress incontinence, the first thing he mentioned was the option of medication. I was a little surprised and then a little impressed. It's amazing to me what they can do with medications.

Because I had only mild stress incontinence, my doctor was sure it could be controlled with medication, so that's the plan we went with and it worked for me."

———————

There are different groups of medications used depending on the patient and the reason for the incontinence.

• Medical Device

"I have been dealing with incontinence since I had my second child. It was one of the more upsetting changes that came from having a baby and it was one I wasn't completely prepared for. I kind of thought all the rumors I heard couldn't be totally true. I was wrong!

My doctor first tried medication, but that didn't work. My incontinence had become too big of an issue. So, he suggested I start doing kegel exercises along with a weight cone. He explained that by doing this, I would strengthen my pelvic floor muscles. By then, I was ready to give anything a try.

So, I continued taking the medication and then I started to do the exercises along with the weight. Things actually did start to get better for me."

———————

There are a few types of surgical procedures that can be used to treat stress incontinence. You will need to discuss the different options with your physician to determine if one of them would be feasible for treating your incontinence.

Many women have benefited from the O-Shot®. For more information, go to **www.totalfemale.com**.

———————

The most important thing to remember from this chapter is simple: it doesn't matter what is causing you to not work down there, you will be able to find a solution. Whether that solution involves medication, exercises, surgeries, creams, or other treatments. You do not have to suffer from urinary incontinence, pain during sexual intercourse, or any other problem that may occur with your genitalia. Please consult with a physician to learn more about your options for treating incontinence.

7

Looking Good – Sometimes a Little Help Doesn't Hurt

"Being self-confident has a positive effect on people's satisfaction with their sexuality and sexual interactions. Pleasurable sexual activities require disclosure of private aspects of the self that people with poor body images are uncomfortable with. People who are discontented with their bodies often experience sexual problems such as the inability to orgasm, while individuals who are comfortable and secure with their bodies often find their sexual experiences more enjoyable and fulfilling." (Importance of Positive Self Image)

The bottom line is it will make you feel good when you are comfortable with the way you look. Unfortunately, we all age and that means skin starts to sag, wrinkles start appearing, blotches come out of nowhere.

There are a few different things in life that can affect sexual desire and on eof those is self-image. When a woman fells like she is getting older and maybe not so attractive anymore, she may find it harder to get turned on.

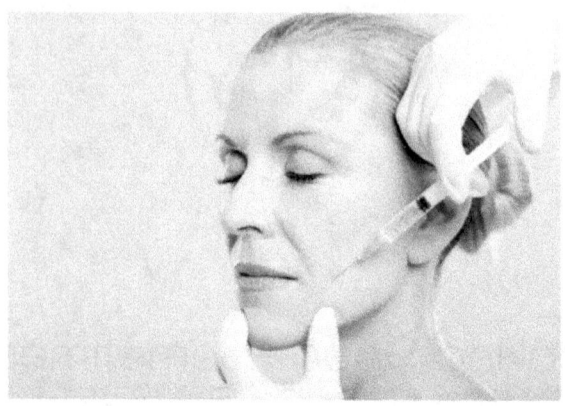

My name is Sonja. I am 49 years old, and up until recently, my age was never of concern to me. Then, I will never forget this day, my husband said "I just love how the corners of your eyes crinkle up when you smile now. It's so cute!"

Oh, no, I thought…if he noticed my crow's feet, what else did he notice? The sagging belly? The way my boobs no longer point up? The ugly brown blotches on the back of my hands? The way things just aren't as …tight…down there? I panicked. My husband meant what he said as a compliment, but it made me realize I just wasn't happy with the way I looked anymore.

Honestly, I just didn't really want to have sex anymore. I was afraid my husband would notice something else sagging. So, I found ways to avoid it. I told him I liked sex with the lights off. I suggested we stay under the covers. I refused to take my top off. It really started to get in the way. I know he noticed too and he did his best to make sure I knew he thought I was sexy. He gave me compliments all the time. But, I didn't see it when I looked in the mirror.

All I could see was this old lady where a young beautiful girl once stood. It was time I did something about it. It was time I got a little help so that I could start liking the way I looked once again.

When you don't think you are pretty or sexy, you will find it much harder to even consider getting turned on. You may avoid sexual encounters altogether, because you don't want your partner or spouse to see you without clothes on.

While there is nothing wrong with aging, there is also nothing wrong with getting a little help with the way you look either. You probably already know about some of the plastic surgeries you could consider, like facelifts, breast augmentation, tummy tucks and Botox injections, all of which can help improve a youthful appearance. So, we won't talk about them in this chapter. Instead, we will discuss some treatments you may not have heard of, such as the Vampire FaceLift® and regenerative hair growth. These types of treatments are designed specifically to reverse the effects of aging!

Vampire FaceLift®

I don't like to look old. I will admit it. Call me superficial if you would like, and I know I am. But, what woman wants to see wrinkles when they look in the mirror? If they were honest with themselves, not a single woman would say they are totally happy with the signs of aging.

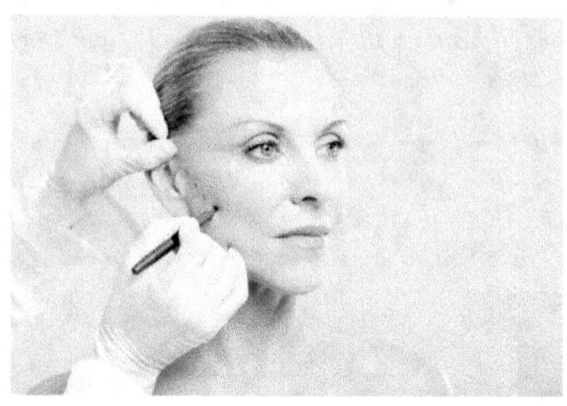

So, when I started to see wrinkles, I panicked. I don't want to look old, for goodness sake! I tried every cream, gel, and masque out there. None of them did a good enough job for me. I still wasn't happy with the way I looked in the mirror.

When I found out about the Vampire FaceLift®, I knew this is something I wanted. It sounded so great since it doesn't even really use anything unnatural. It's my own blood, so it certainly can't be dangerous, I thought. Having the injections done was a piece of cake and I have to say, I am more than happy with the results. Not only did my wrinkles fade, but also my skin just looked younger and healthier. That schoolgirl flush came back when my husband gave me a compliment. I couldn't be happier with the way I look now and I am certainly a tough critic.

When we discussed ways to ensure your vagina stays healthy and you are able to enjoy sexual intercourse, one of the things we mentioned as PRP treatment (platelet rich plasma). This treatment is used in the O-Shot® to rejuvenate the vagina. Now, let's talk about the Vampire

FaceLift®, which uses the same premise to rejuvenate the skin on your face.

What Is It?

As you grow older, several different things happen to the skin on your face:

- Your skin color loses its' healthy look. In fact, it becomes grayer. With less blood flow to the face, the skin essentially begins to starve.

- The skin texture begins to show signs of aging. It doesn't have the same elasticity, so it begins to droop and look tired.

- The actual shape of the face begins to fall in on itself. That's because you lose collagen as you age and your muscles begin to wear out.

These signs are some of the reasons why women are not happy with the way they look. These are also signs that can be rectified with the Vampire FaceLift®.

Many women choose to go in for surgical facelifts, when they don't really need this. That type of surgery is very dramatic and actually involves cutting off skin from the face. It isn't always necessary. Another option many women turn to is filler injections made from hyaluronic acid. The problem with this is the injection is made from chemicals made in a lab. Foreign chemicals will have side effects in the body and could be dangerous in the long term. In addition, the filler injections don't do anything for the texture and color of your skin.

The Vampire FaceLift® is made from platelets in your blood, so it is natural. It will work on all the signs of aging including color, texture, and wrinkles.

How Does It Work?

When we discussed the O-Shot®, we talked about how the platelets work to rejuvenate tissues. When platelets are injected, it is like getting immediate blood flow to the area, drawing more blood and healthier cells. This allows the skin to rejuvenate to the more youthful look, in a more natural manner.

PRP treatments have shown to be so effective that they are used to rejuvenate and heal tissues all throughout the body. For example, when athletes injure their knee or shoulder, PRP injections can help improve and rev up healing.

What Is the Procedure Like?

There are three basic steps to the Vampire FaceLift®. The whole procedure only involves a few needle sticks and no incisions are made at all. In a nutshell, you don't have to worry about the risks that come along with surgery. According to VampireFacelift.com, the steps to the procedure include:

- The procedure begins with safe filler injections.
  These fillers are only temporary and they are used in this case, to create the right shape for the face. It is very important to achieve a natural shape to the face and that's why fillers are used.

The fillers will create a natural shape and this will work sort of as a blueprint for the rest of the procedure.

- Next, the physician will draw approximately two teaspoons of your blood. That's not much at all, but it will be enough to make a big difference. Your blood will go through a spinning process, in a centrifuge, to draw out the platelets. This only takes about 10 minutes, so you don't have to wait long.

The physician then puts the platelets through a process to activate them. This is basically getting the platelets ready to do their healing work and increase blood flow back to the tissue.

- Finally, numbing cream will be applied to your face, so you don't feel the needle stick. Then, a pattern will be used to inject the platelets into the face. Essentially, the platelets in the area will encourage health, blood flow, and growth in the tissue. It will also encourage production of collagen.

In about two or three months, you will see the results of the procedure. Your skin will be healthier. Your face will look younger. You will look and feel younger. The Vampire FaceLift® procedure offers changes that last a minimum of two years.

Recovery

Recovery time from the Vampire FaceLift® is relatively non-existent. You don't have to worry about stitches or anything that will require bed rest. Instead, you can get back to your normal life right away.

By the way, it's called Vampire because it uses your own blood. No Dracula or bat will come out of a cave and suck your blood! It's simply a procedure that understands the power in your own blood and then puts that power to work.

It is important to note that the Vampire FaceLift® isn't for everyone. In some cases, a traditional facelift or other types of injections will be the better option. In fact, the Vampire FaceLift® is not recommended for:

- Women who have fuller faces

- Women who have crepey skin (skin that looks like wadded up paper)

- Women who have very deep wrinkles

It would be very important to discuss your options with your physician before determining if the Vampire FaceLift® is the right option for you.

Regenerative Hair Growth

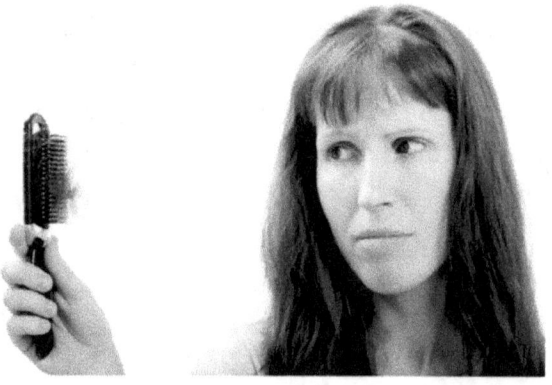

I have never had exactly thick hair, but over the years, I learned all these methods of teasing and combing. I managed to make my hair look much thicker than it really was. It was something I could live with.

When I got pregnant, my hair actually got thicker and I was so excited! It was fantastic how thick and glossy it looked. Then, I had my baby. My hair didn't just go back to being thin. It got worse. The older I get, the worse it gets too.

I am only 45 and you can see my scalp in the front. I hate looking in the mirror. I hate trying so hard to make my hair look thicker and it's just not working. I wear hats so many times just to cover up my bald spot, as I call it.

When I heard about regenerative hair growth, I decided this was certainly something I needed to find out more about.

There are plenty of thinning hair solutions out there. Most of them are geared toward men, but there are options for women. The problem is most of them either don't work so well or end up looking fake. Some of the things you may run across when looking for a solution to thinning hair include:

- Spray on hair

- Hair track implants

- Hair thickening products

- Hair thickening shampoos

Some of these treatments offer varying levels of results, but none of them offer a real solution. That's when regenerative hair growth comes into play. This fairly new solution uses real hair!

"Researchers at Columbia University Medical Center have devised a hair restoration method that can generate new human hair growth, rather than simply redistribute hair from one part of the scalp to another. The approach could significantly expand the use of hair transplantation to women with hair loss, who tend to have insufficient donor hair, as well as to men in early stages of baldness." (Hair Regeneration Method Is First to Induce New Human Hair Growth, 2013)

Standard hair implant procedures simply take tracks of hair from one part of your head (usually around the back of the scalp) and move it to the thinning areas. This is a method of making sure you get to keep your own natural hair. The problem is, you probably don't have enough hair to do the transplant. When your hair thins with age, it thins everywhere, not just on the top like men do.

So, the traditional transplant methods just don't work for women. Regenerative hair growth is different. With this method, doctors can actually grow your own hair. This is done in a couple of different steps. The physician will be able to induce more hair follicles to grow on your head and allow for existing, dead follicles to regenerate.

How It Is Done

Researchers learn how human hair grows now better than ever. One thing they have learned is understand and to better utilize the hair's natural growing patterns. Each hair on your head goes through three phases:

1. Active Growth or Anagen

During this phase, your hair is actively growing. This phase usually lasts around 3 or 4 years or even up to 9 years. However, as women age, this phase becomes shorter. Since fewer hairs are in the active growth phase, the hair will appear thinner.

2. Regressive Phase or Catagen

During this phase, which lasts a few weeks, your hair begins to shed any old strands to make room for new growth. This is why you see hair in your drain or hairbrush. As women grow older, this shedding phase tends to last longer.

3. Resting Phase or Telogen

This phase, which lasts a few months, is when your hair basically goes into hibernation. The hairs don't grow or fall out. They are just there. This phase also gets longer with age.

The degenerative hair growth treatment is done through a process like PRP, which we have already discussed. Through your own platelets and stem cells, the follicles on your head will be healthier and more active.

PRP with ACell®

The PRP with ACell® injection therapy has become one of the leading methods to treat thinning hair on women. Essentially, this uses tissue from your own body to regenerate the follicles and stimulate hair growth. PRP with

ACell® uses adult stem cells, the tissues that are present throughout your body.

In babies and embryos, the stem cells are actively growing and allowing the baby to develop. When you become an adult, the stem cells are inactive. That's why you develop scars when you get a cut or scrape. The body isn't creating brand new tissue, but basically healing over.

The hair regeneration treatment uses adult stem cells that have been reactivated to their original form. Then, the active stem cells, along with the patient's own blood platelets, are injected into the thinning hair area to reactivate the growth of hair from inactive follicles.

Answering Questions about PRP with ACell®

Since this is such a new procedure and you likely did not know much about it before, here are questions you may be asking along with answers to help you better understand the PRP with ACell® procedure.

4. How Long Does the Procedure Take?

You will be given a local anesthetic and then the injections will be placed directly into your scalp. Your physician will need to draw some of your blood to prepare it for the process, but the procedure itself only lasts a matter of minutes.

5. Is It Painful?

Because you are given a local anesthetic, you won't feel much discomfort at all. For a couple of days after the treatment, you may experience mild or moderate discomfort. Your physician will prescribe pain medication to manage this discomfort.

You may see some slight swelling in your forehead along with very slight bruising, but all outward signs of the treatment will disappear in two to three days.

6. How Long Does Recovery Take?

It only takes a couple of days for everything to completely go back to normal. During those couple of days, you likely will not experience anything more than minor discomfort.

7. Do I Have to Take Special Care with My Scalp?

There are no visible signs of the procedure and there will be no scabbing or scarring. You will be able to resume most of your daily activities right away and then you can go back to your normal life in a couple of days.

8. How Long Does It Take to See Results?

You should begin to see new hair growth in about 2 months, with more in 4-6 months and your hair will continue getting new growth for around 12 months. Because this is such a new treatment, there are no long-term studies to determine how long the results from the procedure will last.

9. IS PRP with ACell® Right for Me?

This treatment is good for almost anyone, including women with thinning hair and men who are in early stages of baldness. Because it involves injecting your own blood and cells, it doesn't have any chemical side effects.

The therapy can be used for women and men who have hair loss, people who suffer from alopecia, and people who lose hair in their eyebrows.

If you are experiencing hair loss as you grow older, it is important to note that you don't have to just live with it. Through these new and exciting treatments, using your own cells, you can get thicker, healthier hair, without surgery or using messy creams.

50 Day – 50 LB Weight Loss Program

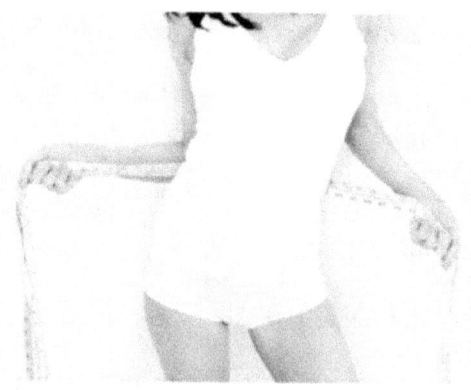

For as long as I can remember, I have struggled with my weight. I guess you could say I am a "curvy" girl. I never minded it, especially when I was a young lady because I had that classic hourglass figure other women envied. As I grew older, the pounds started to add up. Then, by the time I was 45, I looked into the mirror and thought "who is that chubby woman looking back at me?"

It as in that moment, as I stared at a stranger in the mirror, I knew something had to change. I also knew I am not good with waiting. I want to see results fast or I would give up. Yes, I know it's not the best way to be, but I am being honest. We live in a society of instant gratification, and I wanted that gratification for my weight loss. That's why I chose the 50 day – 50 pound weight loss challenge. I figured it would be a great way to shed the fat and get back to my hourglass curves. It definitely worked and I am happy with my body once again.

One of the most frustrating things women may deal with when it comes to their body and physical appearance, is weight. Women have more trouble losing weight quickly than men and as hormones become out of balance, weight loss becomes even more of an issue. If you are experiencing those extra pounds, one thing to consider is the 50 day – 50 pound challenge.

How It Works

First, consult with a physician that specializes in weight loss. They can provide a complete analysis of your health, including your hormone levels, and give you guidance on eating right, exercising and medications.

The 50 day weight loss plan works only if you are committed to losing the pounds. If you aren't committed, you will likely give up and never see the results. So, if you want to make this happen, vow to yourself that you will stick with it. Then follow these steps:

1. Start by weighing yourself. You need to know exactly what you weigh to determine your caloric intake. When you weigh yourself, use a digital scale so that the results will be as accurate as possible.

Additionally, weigh in the morning, before you have eaten anything and without any clothes on.

2. Figure out your caloric intake. Remember that you do not need to starve yourself. It will be counterproductive if you do that. When you starve yourself, you will be likely to binge. Additionally, you will slow down your metabolism and that will make it even harder to lose weight. A physician can help determine your caloric intake.

3. Track everything you eat so that you can make sure you stay in your limits. Remember that you have to include the calories in everything, from salad dressing to cooking sauces to beverages. There are helpful apps you can download on your smart phone to keep up with calories too.

4. Work out! You will need to exercise at least four and preferably five days a week. Your doctor will recommend a program based on your current health situation. You need to exercise in ways that will speed up your heart rate so that you burn more calories. Aerobic exercise should constitute 20 minutes a day for 5 days a week. This can include jogging, swimming, dancing, or kickboxing. Save weight training until you have lost weight, since muscle weighs more than fat.

5. Absolutely, without question, drink eight glasses of water every single day. This will keep your stomach full, so that you don't have snack cravings and it will keep your body hydrated (remember hydration will help with lots of things including vaginal dryness). Drink one glass of water 20 minutes before you eat meals, so that you won't eat as much.

6. Keep a food journal where you can track your exercise, weight loss, and caloric intake. This information will help you stay on track and will give you the motivation to keep going.

7. Cook meals at home, so that you have more control of what goes into them. Cut down calories by using low fat cooking sprays instead of butter. Ensure you are only eating healthy snacks, too. Stick to things like celery and carrots for snacks, so that you won't reach for the junk food.

8. Give yourself a cheat day once every couple of weeks. This will ensure you don't go completely off the wagon and ruin your diet.

If you follow these simple steps, then you should find it easy to drop the pounds quickly. If you don't have that much to lose, then you may have to adjust your caloric intake, so that you do see the results quickly.

Does It Really Work?

This weight loss plan can work, if you stick with it. However, it does require willpower. If you don't stick to a strict caloric intake and if you don't exercise like you should, then you will not be able to drop the pounds.

The 50 day plan can work if you practice self-control. The more you are willing to put into the process, the better the results can be. It really all depends on you and what you are willing to do!

As you age, your physical appearance will change. That doesn't mean you have to look in the mirror and feel old. It certainly doesn't hurt to get a little help. Procedures like PRP treatments can make a drastic difference in what you see when you look in the mirror. If you have an aging face, then you can consider the Vampire FaceLift®. If you have thinning hair, then regenerative hair growth is now available. Thanks to your own blood and stem cells, you can look better and younger without any type of chemicals or surgeries.

Losing weight can help you feel better about yourself as well, and the 50 day plan can make it happen very quickly.

When you feel better about how you look, you will find that this will improve your sex drive too. Self-confidence means feeling good in and out of the bedroom, so you won't have a problem enjoying the sexual side of you.

For more information on a highly successful weight loss program, we recommend the California Medical Weight Management Program. www.calmwm.com

They have treated over 34,000 patients successfully!

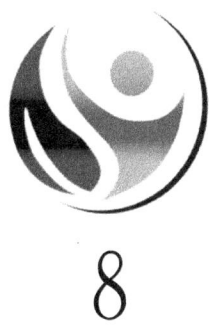

8

Stem Cell Banking

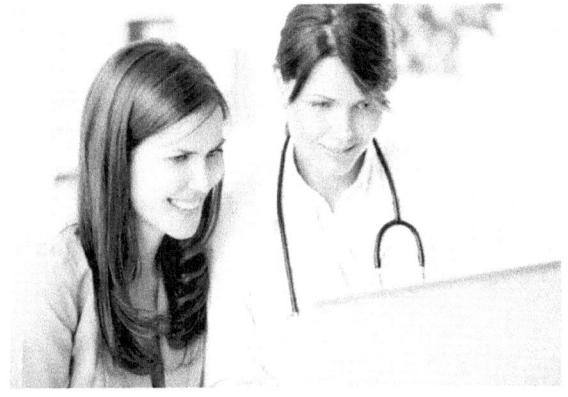

"Stem cells, the precursors to other kinds of cells in the human body, promise near-miracle medical treatments such as regenerating organs and repairing nerves. But stem cell medicine is still in the early stages. Culturing the right kind of cell remains difficult and so far only a few procedures have been FDA approved. Odds are it will be several years before a wide range of ailments can be treated with stem cells.

For those who want to be ready for that day, some companies in the United States are offering people a chance to bank their stem cells for future use." (Emspak, 2013)

The idea of stem cell banking has been catching steam lately, and it is something that you may wish to consider for your own life and future. Let's talk more about this.

What Is It?

Stem cell banking is simply extracting certain cells from your body and then saving them, cryogenically, for future use. It's not a difficult procedure and it doesn't take that much time at all. Quite simply, you will do no more than just give blood. If you have any type of liposuction done, you can even have the stem cells extracted from the fat removed from your body.

In any case, once the physician has your blood, they will be able to extract stem cells that have become deactivated. Then, they will put the cells through a process to reactivate them, so that they become the amniotic cells you had when you were a baby. This way, the stem cells will be ready for use when you need them.

Stem cell banking usually involves a couple of different fees, including:

- An initial fee for collecting and processing your cells. This can cost anywhere between $500 and $8,000.

- A storage fee for cryogenically freezing the cells. This can cost anywhere from $90 to $700, per year, depending on the company that stores your cells.

Importance of It

We have talked about a few different treatments and rejuvenations that can use your stem cells, including the

Vampire FaceLift® and the O-Shot®. Both of these use the cells, and both can be performed at different times in the future. For example, the Vampire FaceLift® will likely wear off several years after you have the initial treatment. Having your stem cells stored makes it much easier to get the treatment again later.

Additionally, stem cells are stronger and more robust the younger you are, so banking them early can be a good idea.

Finally, if we are already able to make your face and vagina look younger with stem cells, imagine what the possibilities may be in the future. It's important to consider stem cell banking now, because you may find the cells you have stored away can be extremely useful in the years to come.

This is just the beginning. There are already research studies in place to determine how stem cells can be used to treat a number of other conditions in the future.

The Future

Now, let's consider all of the things doctors believe stem cells can be used for in the future with more study:

Organ and tissue regeneration	Treatment of angina
Treatment of Alzheimer's	Regenerative treatment of diabetes
Treatment of Parkinson's	Use in cell-deficiency therapy

All of these treatments may be a possibility in the future, but they need more research, since they are largely considered experimental at this time. However, for those people who choose to bank their stem cells now, the treatments available for them in the future may be virtually endless.

For more information on current treatments, research reports; Go to

www.stembanking.com

Risks

Since many stem cell treatments are still in the research phase, the actual risks are in research phases too. There are risks or concerns that have been identified, and it is important that you understand them before you have any procedure:

- A person who has cancer should not be a candidate for stem cell transplants. There is a risk that the disease could be aggravated and may become more aggressive in this case.

- Some disreputable physicians, especially in foreign countries who are charging cheap prices for stem cell procedures, may be doing things that could put you at risk. For example, some doctors have been known to use stem cells from sheep or other types of animals. This could be a very real risk for humans.

If you intend to get a stem cell treatment, then it is absolutely vital that you only do so through a reputable physician, who has the experience, knowledge, and ability to perform the treatment properly. The number one rule you must keep in mind is that this is not something you will want to try to skimp on, just in an attempt to save money. If you do so, you could put yourself at serious risk. If you are considering a stem cell treatment, then here are the questions you can ask a physician to better understand them and what they plan on doing:

- Is this stem cell treatment routine? Has it become a regular treatment or is it in trial phases?

- What benefits can I expect from having this done?

- How long will the treatment take? How long will the results last?

- Where will you get the stem cells for this treatment? Make sure they are only from you!

- How do you go about isolating the stem cells for use?

- How do you go about activating the stem cells?

- How do you know how to identify these cells?

- How do you then deliver the stem cells to my body?

- Do you have the scientific evidence that this procedure has worked?

- Have you done this procedure before? How many times?

- What risks to me come along with this procedure?

- Can I expect any adverse reactions to the procedure?

- What types of follow-up treatments will I need?

- How long will my results last?

- Will you be the doctor doing my treatment or someone else in your office?

- Do you have the credentials to perform this specific treatment (Only approved doctors can do the Vampire FaceLift® and O-Shot®)?

- How much does this treatment cost?

Asking these questions will help you get a better idea of whether or not you have chosen the right physician to perform your therapy, using stem cells.

Aesthetics

There are numerous treatments from stem cells associated with aesthetics specifically, like the Vampire FaceLift® and the O-Shot®. However, as more research is developed in the area of stem cells, the aesthetic uses could continue to grow. Some of the treatments that are already available to make you look and feel younger include:

- Wrinkle treatment on the face, neck, and hands

- Overall facial rejuvenation

- Treatment of the cleavage and chest area

- Filling in volume deficiencies that cause dents in the belly, buttocks, and thighs

- Stimulation of new hair growth on the scalp

- Body contouring treatments for smoother skin on different areas of the body

Stem cells have an extensive rejuvenation effect on almost every part of the body, so that you can look younger, feel younger, and not have to undergo the knife.

Stem cells don't result from some type of chemical treatment you have to put in your body. Often, various surgeries and chemicals can create an unnatural look especially on the face. No one wants to look like they are a plastic doll! Stem cells, which are your own cells, contribute to the growth and rejuvenation of your own cells, tissue, and skin. That means they are completely safe and natural.

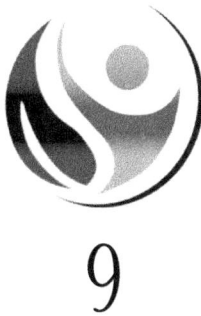

9

Final Thoughts

As a woman, sexuality is a part of your life and it is something that you shouldn't lose just because of age, illness, or body changes. Hormones play a huge role in who you are, controlling your sexuality, sexual drive, and much more. Beyond everything we have talked about so far, there are things you need to consider, so that you can enjoy life to its fullest. Of course, the only way you can enjoy that life is if you are healthy sexually, physically and emotionally.

Things to Address with Him

I love my husband. I really do, and we have a fantastic marriage. We are always open and honest with each other. We communicate well. However, there was one topic I wasn't so good at communicating with him. I didn't know how to tell him that things weren't so good for me sexually.

It's embarrassing to tell someone things like that, even if you have been married for 20 years as we have. For a long time, I just kept it to myself. Then, I realized I was doing him and my marriage a disservice. We both deserved better. So, as hard as it

111

was, I wrote down a list of things I wanted to talk about and then we had a discussion.

He was so supportive. He understood that things were not quite right and he had even known that before I talked to him. He didn't get mad at me or make it all about him. Instead, he said "Ok, honey, what do we need to do?" So, we made a doctor's appointment and found out that my hormones were out of balance.

Once I started taking medication, things started straightening out. Now, my husband and I are more open than ever in the bedroom. I tell him exactly what I want and he tells me what he wants. It's fun and it has even added some spice to our lives.

Talking about things like that was hard. I didn't want to do it, but I am glad I did and I would tell any woman to do the same thing.

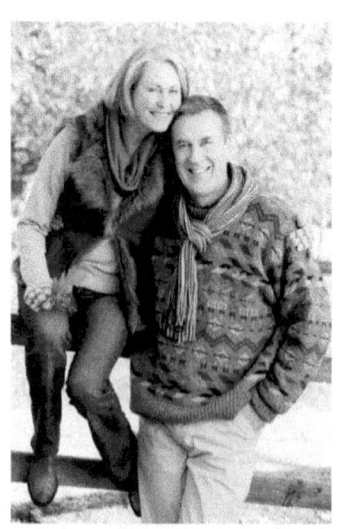

When you are experiencing any problems with your sexual health, it's very important that you talk things over with your partner. If you just stop wanting to have sex, he may have no idea what is going on and he may begin to think he did something wrong. If you and he are open with each other through communication, then there may be changes you could make to improve your sex life.

It's hard to talk about sexual problems though, even if you have been married for decades. You may be shy or you may just be uncomfortable bringing things up. But, when it comes to your sexual health and your sexuality as a couple, talking is a must. To help you out, here are some things you could and should address with him.

The Big "O"

It's common for men to think their ability to get a woman to orgasm as a sign of their masculinity. For that reason, if you no longer achieve orgasm during sexual intercourse, your husband may take it personally. It's very important that you have a discussion with your spouse explaining it has nothing to do with you, but instead about hormonal changes in your body. Some of the things you need to discuss include:

- You are still great in bed. I love sex with you, but one of the side effects of changes in my hormones is inability to climax. Believe me. I want to get back to this, but it has nothing to do with you.

- We may have to try other things that will help me reach orgasms like Scream Cream, so that I have more feeling down there.

- I want to talk to my doctor about my hormonal imbalances. I think if I can get things straight, then I can start climaxing again.

- I can't really climax through penetrative sex right now, but that doesn't mean no pleasure for me. Would you consider direct clitoral stimulation?

Essentially, you want to convey that you do think you may have a problem and you do want to get it fixed, so that you can still enjoy that very special moment during sex with him.

Pain during Sex

Pain during intercourse can be an especially hard topic to bring up, since you have to admit something that he is doing, doesn't feel good. Again, it doesn't necessarily have anything to do with him or his ability to turn you on. If you are dealing with vaginal dryness or you are going through menopause, then you will have more sensitivity in the vaginal area. That means you will have to take extra steps to make sure sex is comfortable.

It's important to address this with your significant other since he may be hurting you without even knowing it. So, some of the things to talk about include:

- It hurts when we have sex because I get dry down there. It has to do with aging and hormones, but it's something we can change.

- Let's start using lubricant. It can even be fun to try a variety of different brands and types to see what we like best. Want to have a little extra fun? We could even try one of the warming types or a flavored one.

- I want to go to the doctor and talk to him/her about the pain I am feeling during sex. It's affecting my sex drive and making me not want to engage in sex even though you do turn me on. I think maybe there is something the doctor will be able to do.

It's good to be open with your spouse. The worst thing you can do is just try to grit your teeth and bear it. By doing that, you will come to fear or resent the very idea of having sex and you may even inadvertently take out that fear or resentment on your spouse. They won't even know what is going on. So, be honest. Tell him what is going on.

Self-Consciousness Issues

When you don't believe you look good, it won't matter what your spouse says about your body. When you stop wanting to have sex, because you aren't comfortable with your body, you will be hurting your relationship with him. Bedroom time is very important to any relationship, so this is something you do need to be open with him abou,t as well. Some of the things to discuss could include:

- I know you think I look good, but I am struggling with my self-confidence right now. I don't like what I see in the mirror. So, be patient with me while I deal with this. Sometimes, I may want to have sex with the lights off or I may prefer to keep my shirt on. Please understand why and allow me do this right now.

- I think I would feel better about myself if I got something done to make my face look younger. I have heard about a Vampire FaceLift®. I think I want to go talk to a physician. Will you support me in this?

115

Again, it's best to just be open and honest. Communication with your spouse and helping them understand what's important to you about your physical appearance, will ensure that the two of you are on the same page.

Even for people who have been married for decades, the sex topic can lead to a difficult discussion. It's embarrassing to talk about problems or issues and it can certainly be hard to explain. However, you probably already know just how important communication is in any marriage, and that communication extends into the bedroom. Tell him what is going on. Chances are he will be more understanding and supportive than you expect.

Knowing That Sex Is Ok after Hysterectomy

This is something that you and your husband should discuss with your doctor. Not everyone understands that it is still possible to have sex, even after a hysterectomy and everything will be normal, for the most part. Once the two of you have communicated and understand that you can still be intimate, keep in mind that lubrication may be more difficult. You may wish to consider a lubricant to make things more comfortable for you.

Knowing When to Talk to a Doctor

> *I knew that in the last few months things have been wrong for me. I couldn't seem to get ...wet anymore when my husband and I fooled around. I had been really tired too. I knew that something was different, but for a long time, I just assumed it was part of aging or maybe that it was some type of phase I was going through.*

So, when things got worse, I realized I should have talked to the doctor in the very beginning. Once I had that conversation with my gyno and found out there were things that could be done, I was glad and I realized there was nothing in the world to be embarrassed about.

I guess I knew something was wrong in the beginning, but I just didn't want to admit it to myself for whatever reason. I wish I had talked to the doctor sooner, but I am glad that I went ahead with the conversation because her treatment suggestions have changed everything for the better.

Often, women overlook hormonal problems simply because they are embarrassed to talk to anyone. Or, they may think "it's just a little twinge" that will eventually go away. So, when should you talk to a doctor?

There are certain signals when you should always talk to a doctor, because you could have a vaginal infection or other condition that could become serious. These issues include:

- If you have sudden pelvic pain or pelvic pain that is severe

- If you feel pain or extreme discomfort in your vagina or labia area

- If you have pain during sex or bleeding after sex

- You never seem to be in the mood for sex and you cannot seem to get turned on

If you have any problems that affect your sex life, from vaginal dryness to pain during intercourse, you need to talk to your doctor right away. You could have an infection or you may have a problem that can easily be managed, with the right medications or treatments.

How to Talk to a Doctor

Of course, knowing you need to talk to a doctor is very different from actually bringing up your sex issues or concerns. Here are some things you can do to get through the conversation, without becoming embarrassed. Remember, that your physician is a professional who has heard virtually anything you could say. They won't judge you or laugh at you. Instead, they will be able to offer solutions that can truly help you. Here are some tips that can help you talk to your doctor with honesty.

- Be prepared. Don't walk in the doctor's office without something written down or arranged. If you don't get prepared, you may forget something or you may get flustered. Before you even go to your appointment, write down a list of questions or things you want to talk about.

- When you make an appointment, mention that you have some things you need to discuss with your physician. This way, the doctor will be prepared for the conversation and will ensure they have enough time to devote to you.

- Don't try to sound super medical. It's better to use your own words to describe your questions or concerns, because you will be able to convey them much more clearly to your physician. If you try to use a lot of medical terms, you may become confused and you may not be able to convey what you want to say.

• Don't save the most important thing for when you get up to leave. Instead, go ahead right at the beginning of the appointment and bring up your sexual concerns. If you wait, your doctor may not have time to answer your questions or address your issues.

• Don't exaggerate or try to downplay your symptoms. Be completely honest with what you tell your physician. They will not be able to diagnose or properly address your condition if you aren't.

• Ask for a referral if needed. There may be times when your doctor is not able to handle the issue, because you will need to see a different kind of physician or specialists. In these cases, ask your doctor for a referral instead of looking for someone on your own.

Preparing for Your Appointment

Make sure you have all of the information your doctor may need. This will include:

• A list of your symptoms – be thorough and honest

• Information on your sexual history – that may include past relationships and past sexual concerns

• A list of questions you would like to ask your doctor

• Information on your medical history – include conditions, medications you take, surgeries, and other things that you have been diagnosed with in the past

Addressing all of your concerns and asking the right questions is an absolute must. Here are some ideas for questions you may wish to bring up with your physician once you have begun the discussion about your sexual problems or concerns:

- What could be causing my problems?

- What types of further testing will be needed to determine what is wrong?

- Do you have a recommended treatment for my condition?

- What are the medications you are prescribing, what do they do and what are their possible side effects?

- What kind of improvement can I expect from the treatment?

- Are there things I can change in my lifestyle to better handle my condition?

- How does my partner need to be involved in my treatment?

- Do you have materials I can take home and study to learn more about my condition?

- Will I have follow up appointments with you or will I need to see a specialist?

- Is this condition long-term or something that will go away with time?

It's ok to ask any questions you may have. The more you ask, the more you and your doctor can thoroughly understand what is going on with you.

Are My Hormones out of Balance?

So, are your hormones out of balance? Only a physician will be able to answer this question thoroughly.

Here are some things to consider. Earlier in this book, we went through lists of specific symptoms of imbalance depending on which hormone was not right. Now, to clarify the issue even more, below you will find a list of statements. Think of those statements as if you are saying them. Answer on a scale of one to five with one being strongly disagree and five being strongly agree. You can even write down this information and share it with your doctor when you schedule an appointment.

- I am tired all of the time.

- I am so tired and exhausted that it interrupts my daily life.

- I wake up in the middle of the nigh covered in sweat.

- Sometimes during the day, I get randomly hot even though the room is cool.

- Before my period, I get extremely moody.

- I have more allergy problems before my period.

- I am asthmatic and I have asthma attacks before my period.

- I just feel down for no reason at all.

- I constantly feel overwhelmed.

- I have gained a lot of weight recently and I don't know why.

- I cannot seem to lose weight no matter how hard I try.

- I have lost a lot of weight recently and I don't know why.

- I do not feel good about myself and the way I look.

- I am not interested in sex anymore.

- I have a lot of trouble with vaginal dryness.

- I experience pain during intercourse.

- I am not able to orgasm anymore.

- My breasts are tender and swollen and I don't know why.

- My period is extremely heavy.

- My period is irregular.

- People around me have noted that I am moody.

- I have trouble with urinary incontinence.

- It's hard for me to concentrate.

Of course, some of these symptoms could indicate something other than hormone imbalance and that's why you need to discuss everything with your physician. However, if you answered three, four, or five on many of these statements, then this could be a good indicator of hormonal imbalance.

A List of Medical Conditions and Treatments That Can Have Sexual Side Effects

No woman on this earth wants to have a mastectomy. In fact, the day I found out I had breast cancer was the worst day of my life. I was terrified. I was so afraid and sad that I cried for about three days straight I think. And, who could blame me? Cancer is a scary thing, and even if the survival rate is high, the treatments themselves can be scary all on their own.

My oncologist explained to me that I would need to go through a series of treatments that would include chemotherapy as well as a double mastectomy. That was the second worst day of my life. After all, my breasts were an essential part of being a woman and they would be taken away. I had no choice though. My cancer was not advanced and since it was confined to my breasts, my doctor felt certain that I would recover and go into remission.

So, after the surgery that took my breasts away and then months of chemo, I got the good news. I was in remission! The cancer was gone. That was certainly one of the best days of my life. Everything would be great now, I thought.

I was 43 years old when this happened. I should add that during that time, my husband of ten years left me. I guess he couldn't deal with the stress of a wife with cancer. That's really neither here nor there though. But, when I had been in remission for about seven months, I met Brad, my now boyfriend.

When Brad and I got serious, I realized something. I was terrified to have sex. I didn't even want to. I had no sex drive and I didn't know if it was because the chemo did something to my hormones or if I was embarrassed to let Brad see me without my shirt on. I thought he would be totally turned off.

I finally sought treatment with my doctor and discovered that I did have a hormonal imbalance. It did have to do with the chemo too. She prescribed medication and that helped things immensely. Then, the day came when things went farther with Brad. I was ready, I thought. I was actually turned on for the first time in more than a year! Then, he reached for the buttons on my blouse and I held my breath. All he continued to tell me was that I was beautiful.

I eventually decided to get reconstructive surgery, but I walked into that surgery with the knowledge that someone thought I was beautiful even without my breasts.

Cancer can wreak havoc on the body. It can ruin hormone balances and destroy self-confidence at the same time. But, all of those things can be treated.

Let's talk about the numerous things that can cause sexual dysfunction in women. Some of them are directly related to hormones, but some actually occur for other reasons. If you are dealing with sexual problems, it is important for you and your physician to pinpoint exactly what is wrong.

- Hysterectomy – There are many reasons why surgery to remove the uterus and possibly ovaries may have to occur. In any case, there are reasons the surgery can have a massive impact on sexual function: you may be self-conscious that your body is different, you may be uncomfortable with any scarring, your hormones will be out of balance if your ovaries are removed, or you may feel less like a woman.

• Mastectomy – If your breasts must be removed due to cancer, this can cause psychological problems that interfere with your sex drive. Breast reconstruction can ease some of this. Additionally, if you had chemotherapy or radiation during cancer treatment, this can have an effect on your hormones and libido as well.

• Extreme Stress, Anxiety, or Depression – If these psychological symptoms are left untreated, this can have a huge impact on your sex drive. Emotional distress can actually interrupt your hormone balance and your monthly cycle.

• Chemotherapy – If you have cancer in parts of your body like the bladder, rectum, ovaries, uterus, or breasts, the chemotherapy can actually cause a myriad of problems. For example, these cancers can actually induce or force menopause, even on a younger woman. The chemotherapy treatments can also lower your libido significantly.

• Cancer – If you develop cancer or other disorders in glands like the adrenal, thyroid, and pituitary, then your hormones can become out of balance, because these glands play such an important role in producing those hormones.

• Antidepressants – Medications called SSRIs or selective serotonin reuptake inhibitors can interrupt the chemicals in your brain that are associated with libido. These medications can include Prozac, Paxil, Celexa, Lexapro, Luvox, and Zoloft.

Note: if you are taking SSRI antidepressants, do not stop taking the medication without the supervision of your doctor. You will need to go through a process to wean your body off of the medication. It can be dangerous to quit cold turkey.

- Antibiotics – These medications kill bacteria in the body, including the good bacteria in your vagina. As a result, you could be more prone to yeast infections that can interrupt your sex life.

- High Blood Pressure Medications – Studies have shown that certain hypertension medications like Prazosin and Clonidine can actually limit or lower the libido.

- Tranquilizers – These medications have been shown to not only limit sex drive, but also make it nearly impossible to achieve orgasm.

- UTIs and Other Infections – Infections of the genital area, such as urinary tract infections, rectal infections, and various vaginal infections can make sex painful. Infections caused by STDs, such as genital warts, can also make intercourse painful.

If you have any of these conditions, discuss your concerns with your physician. There may be different mediations for your condition or there may be specific treatments to restore your sexual function.

10

A Q and A

You may still have questions about your body, your sexual health, your treatment options, and more. Hopefully, by reading the common questions below, you can get the answers that you seek.

When do women normally go through menopause?

The answer can vary from one woman to the next. However, the average age is around 51. At the youngest, some women enter menopause in their mid to late forties while at the latest, some women do not enter until their mid to late fifties.

There have been some cases in which women go through an "abnormal" menopause. In these cases, women may go through this change in their early thirties.

I have never had an orgasm – is something wrong with me?

There is a very high number of women who have never had a climax and many women don't have the ability to orgasm during intercourse. The reasons can vary. For some women, it is a hormonal imbalance and once things are back in balance, the problem could be solved. Some women suffer from psychological issues that keep them from orgasm. Some women simply don't have enough feeling or sensitivity in the clitoris to orgasm. However, there are treatments, which we have discussed. Scream Cream is one of them and medication for hormonal imbalances is another. If you have not had an orgasm or you suddenly cannot climax anymore, talk to your doctor.

I have spotting from time to time. That's normal, right?

No, it isn't. Spotting between your periods is probably an indicator that something may be wrong. It is important that you visit your doctor as soon as possible and discuss this issue with them.

Why do I have major PMS?

Some women think of PMS as a normal part of life, but it actually is a sign of hormonal imbalance. This is especially true if you have serious PMS symptoms. You need to consider whether or not you have other signs of hormonal imbalances and you certainly need to discuss this concern with your physician.

What Is PMDD?

You may have heard of PMDD in reference to more severe PMS. This condition is called premenstrual dysphoric disorder and it can be extremely severe.

> "Premenstrual dysphoric disorder is a severe, sometimes disabling, extension of premenstrual syndrome. Although regular PMS and PMDD both have physical and emotional symptoms, PMDD causes extreme mood shifts that can

disrupt your work and damage your relationships." (Gallenberg)

PMS will often cause symptoms like being emotional, fatigue, experiencing breast tenderness, and having changes in sleep or eating habits. With PMDD, the symptoms are much worse and include one of the following:

- A feeling of sadness or hopelessness

- A strong feeling of anxiety that doesn't go away

- Extreme moodiness to the point that people notice and it damages your relationships.

- Obvious tendency toward anger or irritability

PMDD can be treated and it does need to be treated because it can seriously affect your daily life. PMDD does come from hormonal imbalances and that means hormonal treatments should be considered first. Other treatments include:

- The use of antidepressants. These medications can help reduce the emotional symptoms of PMDD and they can be taken all month or just between ovulation and the onset of your period.

- Birth control pills can be used to even out hormones.

- Some nutritional changes have shown to have an effect on PMDD symptoms. It is important to consume plenty of vitamin B-6, L-tryptophan and magnesium.

Changes in diet should include cutting back on the caffeine and adding more healthy carbohydrates to your diet. It may even help to eat smaller meals throughout the day.

- Some herbal remedies have shown to ease the symptoms of PMS and PMDD. They include chasteberry and supplements using this herb. However, keep in mind that herbal treatments have not been approved by the FDA.

PMDD is not something you should ignore. For that matter, you should not ignore PMS either. Both conditions are symptoms of hormonal changes and imbalances in your body. They can be controlled with the right combination of medications and changes to your lifestyle. So, if you believe you have PMS or PMDD, be sure to discuss this with your physician.

Is there a specific hormone replacement therapy all women should use?

Not necessarily. Different women have different needs and a variety of differences in their bodies. However, bioidentical hormones have shown the most promise for providing the best results. They are natural, so they integrate with the body better and they don't have the side effects of other types of therapies.

You will need to discuss your treatment options with your physician to determine which hormone therapy will work best for you.

Can I still have sex after a hysterectomy?

Yes, you can and you should still be able to enjoy a normal sex life. Some women notice more problems with vaginal dryness after the procedure and you may need to use more lubricant. Additionally, if the hysterectomy involved removal of the ovaries, then you will need hormone replacement therapy.

I heard Vaseline makes a great lubricant. Is that true?

Not really. Vaseline is oil based and it will break down a condom if you use them. It's best to use a lubricant specifically designed for sexual intercourse. Make sure you choose a water-based lubricant, especially if you use condoms.

Won't birth control pills regulate my hormones?

Sometimes and sometimes not. Certain types of birth control pills can have a regulatory effect. However, they also can wreak havoc on your hormones when you stop taking them. It's important for you to discuss your birth control options with the physician and do not depend on the pill solely for the purpose of regulating hormones.

Can I get pregnant after menopause?

After menopause, no. During menopause, yes. Even though your periods will become irregular, there is a good chance you are still ovulating at times and that can mean pregnancy, even if you are 50!

Are stem cells harvested from unborn babies?

There has been controversy about stem cell treatments simply because many of the research studies did use the cells harvested from embryos and fetuses. However, that is not where the stem cells used for your aesthetic treatments will come from. These stem cells are harvested from your own body (adipose tissue, ie..fat) and your own blood. So, if this is an ethical concern to you, you can rest assured that you will not have to deal with a moral dilemma.

Can Viagra® work for women?

Women have often wondered why there isn't a Viagra® for them and they may even wonder if they could use the little blue pill themselves. However, there hasn't been much studied about this and no one knows what side effects it may have. There is no FDA approval and the side effects can be very unpredictable. Viagra® is only available by prescription to men or through illegal channels on the Internet. The problem with those illegal channels is that you will have no way of knowing what you actually are taking or even if it has any Viagra® in it. It is not worth the risk.

I am pregnant. My friends told me my hormones would go back to normal after the baby is born. Is that right?

Normally, your body will begin to straighten out in the months after you have the baby. However, this is not always the case. Some women continue to have hormonal problems for many years afterward.

If you have any reason to believe your hormones are not right or that they are not getting better, then consider talking to a doctor. You may need treatment to get everything working properly again.

Am I crazy for wishing I had never had a baby? (my little girl is 2 weeks old and I love her to pieces)

Many women suffer from something called post-partum depression. This is a case of severe depression, due solely to a severe imbalance of hormones in your body after childbirth. The answer to the question is that you are not crazy. Post-partum depression is both normal and not normal at the same time. It's normal in that many women suffer from it, so you are not alone. It is not normal in that it indicates a severe hormone imbalance.

If you feel depressed, sad, resentful, detached, and extremely tired all the time, right after having a baby, discuss your concerns with your doctor. You are not a bad mother for having those thoughts. You are simply dealing with a hormone imbalance that can be corrected.

I can't imagine letting someone put a needle down there. Doesn't it hurt?

Obviously, women who are considering an O-Shot® will be concerned about the needles in such a sensitive place. Keep in mind, though, that a local anesthetic will be used. At most, initially you may feel a small amount of minor discomfort.

Is vaginal dryness always a sign of unbalanced hormones?

In one way or another, yes. Vaginal dryness may be indirectly caused by chemotherapy or radiation, medications, and certain other treatments. However, the direct cause will be hormones. The cancer treatments may damage your body's ability to create estrogen. The same is true of medications and certain medical treatments. When you aren't producing enough estrogen, then you will experience vaginal dryness, among other symptoms.

What if my incontinence cannot be treated with medications?

As we discussed earlier, there are actually numerous different treatments available for incontinence depending on the type of problem you have. The O-Shot®, medical devices, creams, and even surgery can be used to treat the condition. Even if medication doesn't seem to be working, don't assume that nothing can be done. You will need to discuss each type of treatment option with your doctor to determine which will work best for you.

I don't understand. How do hormones in my brain affect my sexuality?

That can be a little confusing, but keep in mind that your whole body works together to function properly. The hormones that the glands in your brain produce, will regulate what other parts of your body do. Hormones are like messengers or couriers, that carry messages and directives all throughout the body.

So, when hormones in your brain tell your ovaries and uterus to get to work, then your body will go through the process of your menstrual cycle.

In other words, if hormones in your brain do get out of balance, then this can affect your menstrual cycle, as well as your sex drive. Your body really does work together in this way.

Is it ever normal for sex to hurt?

Unfortunately, many women think that sex will hurt sometimes. But, that isn't the case. If sex hurts for you, then something is wrong. It's important that you address this issue. We have discussed some of the causes of sexual pain already in this book, but let's run through them one more time:

- Quick developing pain during sex could indicate an infection. Some infections include vaginitis, warts, or genital herpes.

• Lack of lubrication can be responsible for pain during sex, especially if it feels like something is chafing or burning at your vaginal entrance.

• Vaginal inflammation can be responsible for pain during sex as well. If you have an inflammation, such as a yeast infection, this could be the cause of the discomfort.

• You could have a benign cyst on the Bartholin's gland. This can cause severe pain during sex.

• Ovarian cysts can cause pain during sex, especially during deep penetration. Other pain from deep penetration could be caused by a retroverted uterus, pelvic inflammatory disease, or abdominal adhesions.

If sex hurts for you, it is extremely important that you discuss this with your doctor. This is not normal and it is not something that you should continue to deal with.

Could a hormonal imbalance cause bad skin and dry hair?

This is a very common symptom of a malfunctioning thyroid. When your thyroid is not producing hormones correctly, you may experience very poor, dull or lifeless skin, as well as hair that just looks dull and flat. You may also notice that your fingernails are very soft and tear very easily.

If you are experiencing other signs of a hormone imbalance and you have poor skin, hair, and nails, then it would be a very good idea to schedule an appointment with your doctor. Your physician may feel that a thyroid test is in order.

It's ok to have questions. You should want to know more about your body and your sexuality. In fact, if you still have questions even after reading this, then it is important that you write them down. Then, when you visit your physician, you can discuss those questions and then get the answers that you need. Never leave a question unanswered when you are talking about your body. If you don't understand something, you may be dealing with a condition or an imbalance that could be treated very easily.

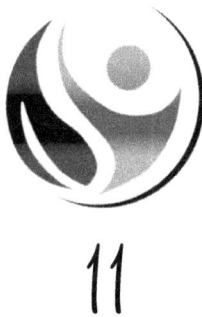

11

Seeking Help - Sex Therapy

Having discovered you may have a sexual problem, the first question you need answered is whether the symptoms you may be experiencing have a medical cause. If there is any possibility of a medical problem, always start by consulting your physician or a medical specialist. You may discover that your symptoms aren't medically orientated, or that in addition to a medical issue, your problem requires psychological help. In most cases self-help will not be enough. Many sexual problems require professional help by a clinician, trained in sex therapy.

Sex therapy, like most forms of therapy, is designed to be both a healing and a growth process. Sex therapy focuses on the sexual problem, as opposed to anxiety, depression, or stress. The client is looking for treatment that is designed specifically to correct their individual sexual problem. Sex therapy doesn't focus solely on sex. Our sexuality is a big part of our lives, making it impossible to focus on sex alone. It is impossible to have an understanding of your sexuality, without taking into consideration your upbringing, religious beliefs, health, relationships, self-esteem, psychiatric status, and more. Sex is such an important part of our lives, it is hard to talk about any of these topics, without also talking about sex.

The sex therapist may treat you individually, with your partner or in a group, based on your needs. A Sex therapist usually begins with a review of your upbringing, relationships, and current level of adjustment. The sex therapist will make suggestions about what factors may be contributing to your sexual symptom and, more important, what steps can help resolve the difficulty. Most therapists focus on quality of life, preferring to work toward helping you realize your potential to live and love most fully. A sex therapist will approach the problem as a shared opportunity for you (or the couple) to discover ways of increasing emotional and physical intimacy. You (or the couple) will be encouraged to find pleasure in your sexuality and become comfortable giving and receiving pleasure. The treatment will include identifying and examine feelings, gaining insight into reasons of behavior, improving communication, learning new ways to approach problems and building up strengths.

Most clients do not know what to expect in sex therapy. Be assured that in legitimate sex therapy, you will not be asked to take off your clothes, have sex with your partner in front of the therapist, or have sex with the therapist. You should, at all times, feel that you are being treated in a professional manner and that your values and religious beliefs are respected.

The length of treatment can vary depending on the individual or couples needs, and can range from a couple of visits to many months of weekly sessions. Your sex therapist should be able to give an estimate of the number of sessions required to accomplish treatment goals. Many sex therapists will assign "homework" to help the couple discover patterns in their sexual relationship, and help the couple learn and practice new practices. The sex therapist will encourage the couple to be honest about their needs and frustrations within their relationship; as well as looking at how they relate to each other. This will help the couple discuss the struggles they are having, as well as the reasons for avoiding intimacy.

When finding a sex therapist, you want to look for a skilled mental health professional who has additional training and experience in the area of human sexuality. You can obtain a list of certified sex therapists in your area by visiting AASECT's website at www.aasectorg. There are also many excellent sex therapist who do not have a formal certification, but are well trained and highly experienced in treating sexual problems. You can ask your healthcare provider if he or she can recommend a qualified sex therapist. You may also contact the psychology or social work department at your local university and ask for recommendations. In addition, contact your state psychological association, psychiatrist association, or the state office for the National Association of Social Workers (NASW) for recommendations. Check the yellow pages under psychologists; counselors; or marriage, family, child, and individual counselors and look for therapists who specialize in treating sexual problems. Or you can simply type in "sex therapy" into any popular search engine.

Once you have a therapist, call and ask questions before scheduling your first appointment. Find out about the therapist's training and their experience in treating sexual problems. Ask about the cost of therapy and whether the therapist accepts insurance. If the therapist is unwilling to answer these basic questions, you may want to keep searching. As a client, you have the right to know what kind of services you're purchasing.

What do you want in a sex therapist? People often wonder whether they should see a female or male therapist. Research shows that sex therapy can be effective regardless of the therapist's gender. You always want to feel comfortable meeting with your therapist. You need to be able to trust your therapist and believe that he or she is concerned about your well-being and is respectful of your circumstances, feelings, and beliefs. After a few sessions you are still uncomfortable discuss your concerns. If you still feel uncomfortable, consider transferring to another therapist. Be careful that by changing therapists, you're not "shooting the messenger." To grow you will likely have to face things that will make you feel uncomfortable. It can be tempting to blame the therapist for this discomfort, rather than asking what it is about yourself, your background, or your relationship that Insight be creating this discomfort. If you want to change therapists, be sure that you're reacting to just bad chemistry and not being uncomfortable with the pain and embarrassment that are coming from the truth.

If you develop a sexual problem it should not be ignored. Sexual Problems can affect our self-esteem, Place a strain on our relationships, and, in some cases, serve as a warning for undiagnosed medical problems. For these reasons, Medical and psychological help are available and highly effective. Reading this book can be an important step in overcoming a sexual problem. We encourage you to take as many additional steps as necessary to continue your journey to sexual health and satisfaction.

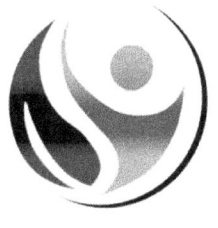

Conclusion

You are a woman. You are a sexual woman. You shouldn't have to deal with sexual dysfunction, no matter the reason for it, without some type of treatment or change in your life. People may tell you that sexual changes are normal. They may even try to say changes are just a part of life. This just isn't the case.

Sexual dysfunction can be caused by a variety of different reasons, but more often than not, hormones are the culprit. Since there are so many reasons why your hormones can get out of balance, this can be a problem for women of many different ages. As we have discussed throughout this book, you could face hormonal imbalances that cause sexual problems from:

Illness or injury	Prolonged psychological conditions
Menopause	Malfunctioning glands
Childbirth	Pre-menopause

It doesn't matter which of these categories you fall into, you deserve a healthy sex life. It is a part of a healthy life overall. With the right treatments, and there are certainly cutting edge options available, you can enjoy a restored hormonal balance and a restoration in your enjoyment of sex.

Understanding your sexual health is an absolute must. That is the only way you will be able to notice if something is wrong or off. If you don't know your body, things could be changing and you may be completely oblivious, until the issue gets out of hand.

Hopefully, through this guide, you have become familiar with the conditions that could affect your body, but more importantly, you have become more familiar with you.

Now, go out there and be the happy, healthy, and sexual you that you are.

For more in depth information on hormones

My Hormones; A simple guide to better and longer living
By; Mark Weis, MD and Douglas Ginter
www.myhormones.com

For more information on Men's Sexual Health.

Total Male; Saving your life by taking charge of your sexual health
By: Mark Weis, MD and Douglas Ginter
www.totalmale.com

For more information on Female's Sexual Health

www.totalfemale.com

For the men in your life

www.totalmale.com

Works Cited

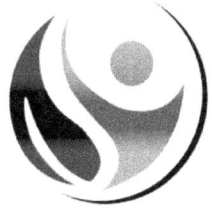

Edmonds, M. (n.d.). *How Vaginas Work*. Retrieved June 17, 2014, from How Stuff Works: http://health.howstuffworks.com/sexual-health/female-reproductive-system/vagina2.htm

Emspak, J. (2013, June 12). *Bank Your Stem Cells for Future Use*. Retrieved June 23, 2014, from Discovery News: http://news.discovery.com/tech/biotechnology/bank-your-stem-cells-future-use-130612.htm

Freeman, S. (n.d.). *What Happens in the Brain During Orgasm?* Retrieved June 17, 2014, from How Stuff Works: http://health.howstuffworks.com/sexual-health/sexuality/brain-during-orgasm2.htm

Gallenberg, M. (n.d.). *What's the Difference between Premenstrual Dysphoric Disorder and Premenstrual Syndrome*. Retrieved June 24, 2014, from Mayo Clinic: http://www.mayoclinic.org/diseases-conditions/premenstrual-syndrome/expert-answers/pmdd/faq-20058315

Hair Regeneration Method Is First to Induce New Human Hair Growth. (2013, October 21). Retrieved

June 20, 2014, from Newsroom Columbia University: http://newsroom.cumc.columbia.edu/blog/2013/10/21/hair-regeneration-method-is-first-to-induce-new-human-hair-growth/

Importance of Positive Self Image. (n.d.). Retrieved June 20, 2014, from SOC: http://www.soc.ucsb.edu/sexinfo/article/importance-positive-self-image

It's All about Balance. (n.d.). Retrieved June 18, 2014, from Connections Women's International: http://www.womensinternational.com/all_about_balance.html

Jackson, R. (n.d.). *Progesterone Creams.* Retrieved June 18, 2014, from How Stuff Works Health: http://health.howstuffworks.com/wellness/natural-medicine/alternative/progesterone-cream1.htm

Kuzmarov, I. (2008, August). *Sexuality and the Aging Couple.* Retrieved June 19, 2014, from Medscape: http://www.medscape.com/viewarticle/586758_2

Normal Menstrual Cycle. (n.d.). Retrieved June 17, 2014, from WebMD: http://www.webmd.com/women/tc/normal-menstrual-cycle-topic-overview

Pappas, S. (2011, August 3). *Nipples 'Light Up' Brain the Way Genitals Do.* Retrieved June 15, 2014, from Live Science: http://www.livescience.com/15380-nipples-genitals-brain-map.html

Scream Cream. (n.d.). Retrieved June 20, 2014, from IJPC: http://www.ijpc.com/_pdf/Scream_Cream.pdf

Sexual Difficulties. (n.d.). Retrieved June 14, 2014, from Women's Health: http://www.womenshealth.gov/aging/sexual-health/sexual-difficulties.html

Streicher, L. (2014, March 19). *Pain or Pleasure? The O-Shot®.* Retrieved June 19, 2014, from Oz Experts: http://blog.doctoroz.com/oz-experts/pain-for-pleasure-the-O-Shot®

Tension Free Vaginal Tape for Stress Incontinence in Women. (n.d.). Retrieved June 19, 2014, from WebMD : http://www.webmd.com/urinary-incontinence-oab/tension-free-vaginal-tape-for-stress-incontinence-in-women

The Hormone Diet. (n.d.). Retrieved June 18, 2014, from WebMD: http://www.webmd.com/diet/hormone-diet

Vampire FaceLift® Procedure Explained. (n.d.). Retrieved June 20, 2014, from Vampire FaceLift®: http://vampirefacelift.com/

What Are Pheromones? Do Humans Have Pheromones? (2011, August 11). Retrieved June 17, 2014, from Medical News Today: http://www.medicalnewstoday.com/articles/232635.php

Women's Health. (2012). Retrieved June 16, 2014, from WebMD: http://www.webmd.com/women/picture-of-the-breasts

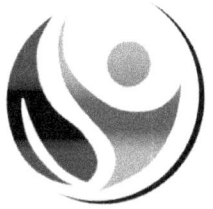

About the author

Douglas Ginter has over twenty years' experience in the health care industry. The former CEO of an FDA-licensed pharmaceutical manufacturer located in Orange, California, Ginter is CEO of multiple companies, including Prescription Headquarters, a compounding pharmacy; Physicians Professional Laboratory, a CLIA certified laboratory; and Physicians Products, a physician's management company. He is also co-creator of the Clearly Beautiful line of cosmetic products used exclusively by dermatologists and plastic surgeons.

Mr. Ginter, co-author with Dr. Weis of *My Hormones: A Simple Guide to Better and Longer Living,* also *Total Male: Saving Your Life By Taking Charge Of Your Sexual Health,* is a member of American Academy of Anti-Aging Medicine, American Pharmacists Association, California Pharmacy Association, and the International Academy of Compounding Pharmacists.

Jason Sachman, MD grew up on the north side of Chicago before completing his undergraduate education with a Bachelor of Science in Psychology and Biology at The University of Texas, Austin. He then returned home for his doctorial degree at **The Chicago Medical School.**

Dr. Sachman went on to residency training at **Loma Linda University Medical Center in Orthopedic Surgery.** He has a background in concierge style medicine and believes this is an essential way to place each patient at the center of his own care. This allows enormous focus and attention to be placed on the specific healing needs of each unique individual.

Since becoming involved in the wellness and anti-aging medicine, Dr. Sachman has taken an interest in treating the entire body and mind. He believes harmony and health throughout all systems are key to enjoying optimal performance and longevity. That is why restoring hormone balance is the forefront of his concern for wellness; because hormones impact so my vital functions in the body and also the brain that may directly relate to maintaining a youthful spirit and essence. Dr. Sachman understands that as we live longer and stronger, quality of life and prevention of both mental and physical disease and deterioration must become a greater focus as we pioneer into a new age of medicine. Jason Sachman is the medical director at Total Medical Center in San Jose, CA. **www.totalmedicalcenter.com.**

www.ingramcontent.com/pod-product-compliance
Lightning Source LLC
Chambersburg PA
CBHW070656290526
45790CB00001B/337